Black Seed

Oil Master

Guide Book

""

Black Seed Oil Master Guide Book

Pixie Seymour

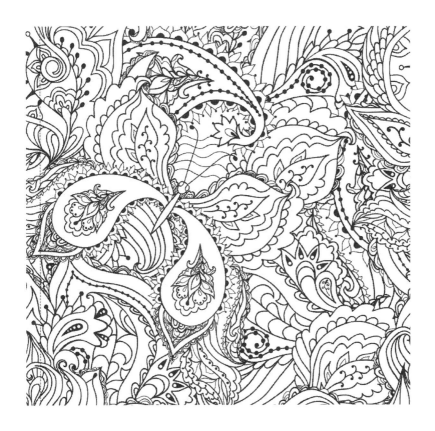

Copyright

ISBN-13: 978-1984034335
ISBN-10: 1984034332

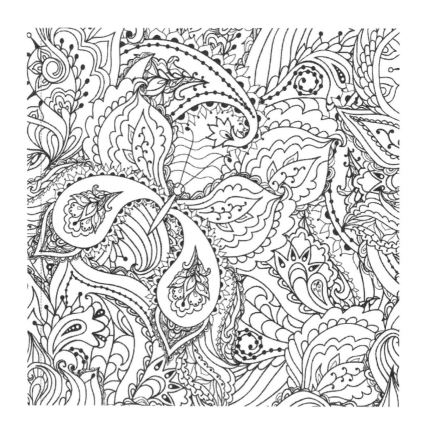

Dedication

I wouldn't be on this earth if it wasn't for my beloved children, so again, I am dedicating this book to all four of them; Moo, Buzz, Boo and Possum. I love you all so much it defies words! Mwah!

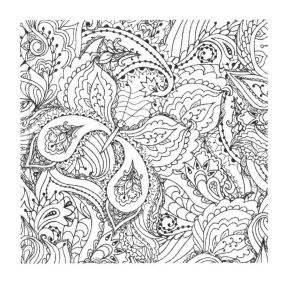

Table of Content

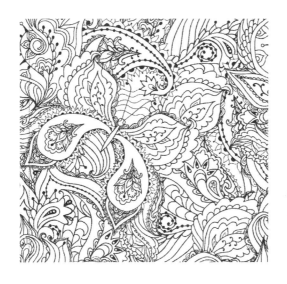

Preface

In this book, I am going to explore the scientific research and the anecdotal evidence for the amazing properties of black seed oil. For ease of reference, I have sorted this book into ailments assisted and they are alphabetically organized.

Black seed oil has been known throughout history as a cure for all ailments except death. I really think this underrated little seed oil is worthy of your attention, even if only ever used as a daily tonic.

Before we go any further, I should point out that I am NOT in any way medically qualified, unless you count 10,000+ hours of research as being qualified. Any and all so-called alternative treatments should be thoroughly researched and run past your doctor before you use them. Do I do that?

Well, no I don't. I offer myself as a guinea pig for many natural treatments and I rarely to never attend an allopathic doctor. Why? Because my thinking is that Mother Nature was right long before modern medical doctors had their chance to experiment on us. However, I cannot recommend that you do the same, because, other than potentially getting myself in trouble with the law, how could I possibly know what is best for you?! I cannot. So, I do not ever recommend any course of action for anyone else, I just put forward my research.

My aim in writing this guide is to help you start to understand just how wildly healthful black seed oil is for the human body. You can read this book from cover to cover, or just skip to the section you're most interested in, then you can come back later to read the lot or just keep as a reference book.

The list of ailments that black seed oil has been known to help with is as long as your proverbial arm. This oil certainly has a big reputation and, in my research travels, I have discovered that its fantastic reputation is very well founded.

I've covered dozens of ailments in this book and I'm sure there will be more in the future with the intense amount of interest this wonder oil is generating.

Book Organization

I had written 20 chapters when it suddenly occurred to me to ask people what ailments they'd like included in the book. I asked my friends what they would like included and another 8 chapters were born! My heartfelt gratitude is included in the acknowledgements.

Throughout the chapters, I've included the references to the scientific papers I'm referring to at the end of each chapter, so you can go read these research papers for yourself.

Far be it for me to tell you what to do with your own body. This book is about *me* handing *you* the reins to becoming your own health advocate.

Enjoy!

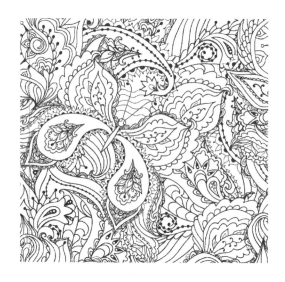

Acknowledgements

Thank you to all those that have helped me in this, my 3rd book project.

It's impossible to track just who sparked what ideas in my brain, but everyone I interact with has a puzzle piece for me, and for that, I thank you all! What I *can* do is thank those who helped me forge the content by answering my call for additional chapters. They are listed in order of suggestion made...

Thank you, Vicki R. for the suggestion of colds/flu and the immune system and, another thank you to you, Vicki, for the other suggestions of gut health and 'Is it safe for children?' Thank you, Constance N. for the suggestion to include a section about reputable suppliers. I have run protocols on myself with 7 different oils, so yes, I have now included the run-down on which is what in regards to quality, taste and availability. Because website links change all the time, I am including the links to suppliers on my website at; www.detoxnanturalliving.com

Thank you to Sue M. for the suggestions to include epilepsy, tumour shrinkage (aside from cancer) and parasites.

Thank you to Anita A. for suggesting for me to include instructions on making black seed oil at home. Trusted organic suppliers have also been included in the references section, on multiple requests.

Thank you to Judy C. for the suggestion to include thyroid. Another body 'control' centre well worth keeping healthy!

Thank you to Tj F. for the suggestion to include the rewiring of the brain after drug withdrawal reference. Much appreciated, dear Tj, and thank you for your friendship.

Thank you to my dear Friend, Josephine A. for putting forth fibromyalgia as a research point. Dear Lady, it is my pleasure to bring you this information. Thank you also, to the lovely Leona W. for also suggesting fibromyalgia.

My acknowledgements wouldn't be complete without thanking my dear friend, Able. He allows me to continue to wear my rose-coloured glasses while enabling me to write my books. So, thank you. All of us girls love you dearly.

Last but not least, I'd like to thank my dear dogga, Lulu. Her attention seeking behaviour every hour or so kept me moving around often, despite sitting on my backside for months writing. Thank you, dear dogga!

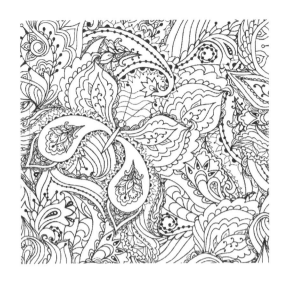

About Black Cumin

"I thought it was good" is the understatement of next year!

Black seed is also known as Barakat, Black coriander, Black cumin, Black seed, Charnuska, Cheveux de Vénus, Cominho Negro, Cumin Noir, Rennel flower, Fitch, Graine de Nigelle, Graine Noire, Habbatus sauda, Kalajaji, Kalajira, Kalonji, La Grainer Noire, Love in a Mist, Mugrela, Nielle, Nigella sativa, Nigelle Cultivée, Nigelle de Crête, Nutmeg Flower, Poivrette, Roman-Coriander, Schwarzkummel, Small Fennel, Toute Épice, Upakuncika.

Arabic: Habatut Barakah Shooneez or Habba Sauda, Habb al-barka
Chinese: Hei Zhong Cao Zi or Pei hei zhong cao

About Black Cumin

Sankrit: Krishana – Jiraka, Upakunchika

German: Schwarzkümmel

French: Cheveux de Vénus, Nigelle

Hindi: Kalonji.

Marathi: Kalonji Jire

A member of the Ranunculaceae family, this little seed has been used since antiquity with the first mention noted in 1025A.D. in 'The Canon of Medicine' by Ibn Sina.

Being the most researched plant in science, and mentioned in the Qu-ran and the King James Version of the Christian bible, black cumin (Nigella sativa) has been aiding human beings for many thousands of years. Just because modern medicine has all but ignored it in favour of big pharma 'quick fixes' doesn't mean we should ignore its benefits.

To the Ancients of many different traditional forms of medicine such as Ayurveda, Unani-Tibb and Siddha, this little black seed of goodness is a medicine gift from God. To modern medical researchers, this is a wonder of Nature. Whichever way you look at it, black cumin has been saving lives well before the first allopathic pill was ever produced.

Black seed oil is ranked very highly among the world of herbal plants. In regards to the sheer volume of research that has been performed upon it, Nigella sativa is the most studied plant we've ever known. Scientists have been looking at Nigella sativa as a medicinal treatment for decades, but it's only during the last few years that we, the public, are beginning to hear about it.

The Greek physician, Dioscorides, used Black cumin seed to treat nasal congestion, headaches, intestinal parasites and toothache.

Hippocrates himself regarded Nigella sativa as an extremely valuable remedy in liver and digestive disorders.

Chemical Composition

The basic chemical composition of black cumin oil has been very heavily researched over the last few decades.

Black seed oil owes a lot of its freakish healing abilities to its most active ingredient, Thymoquinone (TQ). Other active components in black seed oil include:
- 6-methoxy-coumarin
- 7-hydroxy-coumarin
- Alpha-hedrin
- Arvacrol
- Carvacrol
- Dithymoquinone
- Essential amino acids
- Essential fatty acids
- Flavonoids

- Nigellimine
- Nigellicine
- Nigellidine
- Oxy-coumarin
- Thymohydroquinone
- Steryl-glucoside
- Tannins
- Thymol
- Thymoquinone

There are 15 amino acids found in black cumin seed oil and 9 of those are essential amino acids which are:
- Methionine
- Histidine
- Isoleucine
- Leucine
- Lysine
- Threonine
- Tryptophan
- Phenylalanine
- Valine

Nigella sativa increases the antioxidant activity of the following enzymes:
- Catalase
- Glutathione peroxidase
- Glutathione-s-transferase)

Making it even more of a scientific wonder, black seed oil

also contains:
- Sodium
- Potassium
- Beta-carotene
- Ascorbic acid
- Quercetin
- Luteolin
- Arginine
- Folic acid
- Calcium
- Vitamin B1, B2 and B3
- Iron

23 Pharmacological Actions (That We Know Of!)

Pharmacological action = description of how a chemical will behave in the body or in the environment.

Yet another reason why black cumin is such a powerful gift from Nature is the wide array of pharmacological actions it displays. It almost seems like it 'reads' a given environment and morphs into whatever that environment needs in order to get back to balance. This is truly a gift from Nature/God/whatever you want to call the phenomenon that gave us everything we need in abundance and in Nature. We are of the Earth and so it seems a logical conclusion to make to think that our healing will also be of the Earth. Black cumin seed demonstrates my point exactly. Welcome to the most healing substance we have!

Pharmacological Actions of Black Cumin:
- Anti-diabetic
- Antibacterial
- Anti-cancer
- Anti-convulsant
- Anti-fungal
- Anti-inflammatory
- Anti-microbial
- Antioxidant
- Anti-oxytocic
- Anti-schistosomiasic
- Analgesic
- Bronchodilator
- Cardiovascular-protective
- Contraceptive and anti-fertility
- Gastro-protective
- Hepato-protective
- Immunomodulator
- Nephro-protective
- Neuro-pharmacological
- Pulmonary-protective
- Renal-protective
- Spasmolytic
- Testicular-protective

There aren't many physical issues that black cumin seeds cannot help the body beat. With pretty much zero side effects in therapeutic doses and the healing superpowers of black seed oil, it's gobsmacking that most of the Western world hasn't heard of it yet!

Once I started researching, I was amazed, and still am, at the wide array of health conditions that this cute little black seed helps us with.

Dosage

I pay black seed oil its due respect like other powerful substances. Therefore, when I first got it, I tried a single drop on my wrist. When I had no reaction to that, I tried a couple of drops. Then a few drops in my mouth and gradually moved up to the dosage I use now. It's just the sensible thing to do. In addition, I only dose on a daily protocol with black seed oil for about 1-2 weeks at a time. Then I give my liver a break and stop taking it for a while. Always give the oil a helping hand to move through your body with a glass of water to wash it down.

Is it Safe?

I found a few research projects that assessed the safety of black cumin seed on humans and animals. I couldn't find research to suggest that black cumin seed is dangerous. In fact, the opposite is true; it's generally very safe even in moderate to high doses if you also protect your liver with plenty of water and don't high dose for extended periods of time unless you are following a health care provider's plan for chronic illness.

Research

I found numerous studies suggesting that black seed oil has a very high safety margin.

"'Median Lethal Dose' (MLD or LD50) is a medical research term that describes the situation of half the test subjects dying of the substance being tested. In 2008, researchers found that the LD50 for mice and rats after oral ingestion was 870.9 mg/kg. To put that in perspective, 870.9mg per kilo of body weight is the lethal dose, so for a human weighing 70kg, the lethal dose would be 60963mg. The LD50 values presented here are 10-15 times and 100-150 times greater than doses of Thymoquinone reported for its anti-inflammatory, antioxidant and anti-cancer effects" REF - 'Oral and intraperitoneal LD50 of Thymoquinone, an active principle of Nigella sativa, in mice and rats' https://www.ncbi.nlm.nih.gov/pubmed/19385451

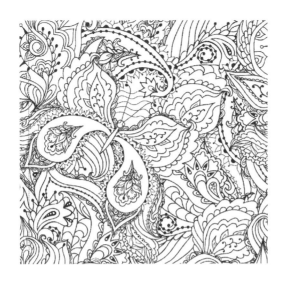

Chapter 1 – Acne and Eczema

I have grouped acne and eczema together because they are both skin conditions, even though they are caused by different underlying factors. Both result in an on-skin inflammatory response.

Acne

Acne can result from a combination of conditions that can and often do persist for many years after the normal teenage 'pimply' time ends. By the time you emerge from that stage of life, if you still have acne, then you really ought to be getting onto a black seed oil supplement protocol if you can.

Black cumin oil has a natural anti-histamine, which is great for treating the inflammation associated with acne.

What Is Acne?

"Propionibacterium acnes is a gram-positive human skin bacteria that can survive without harming its host, that prefers anaerobic growth conditions and is involved in the pathogenesis of acne."

(Anaerobic means "living in the absence of oxygen", so it stands to reason that giving this bacteria oxygen would also help to get rid of acne.)

This skin condition can be caused by an array of different inter-reacting factors, for example:

- Hormonal levels
- Dietary intake
- Skin inflammation
- Infections
- Damaged skin
- Poor nutrition

Usually, at about 1-3 years prior to puberty, the Propionibacterium acne bacteria colony begins. During this time, numbers of P acne rise from fewer than 10 per square centimetre to about 106 per square centimetre! "Mainly found on the face and upper throat, the P acne grows in the lipid-rich micro-environment of hair follicles. The P acne produces inflammatory responses that result in acne pustules, papules, and nodulocystic lesions i.e. breakouts." REF - 'Propionibacterium Infections'

Help for Acne Scars

Black seed oil helps reduce infections and fungal growths on the skin.

There was a study in 2010 using a 10% topical lotion which found a "93% good to moderate improvement in papules and pustules after 2 months"

The inflammatory and antioxidative activities of the active ingredients in black seed oil are an excellent catalyst for reducing acne scarring too.

"In a clinical study, N. sativa oil lotion 10% significantly reduced mean lesion count of papules and pustules after 2 months of therapy.

In the test group, the response to treatment was graded as good in 58%, moderate in 35% and no response in 7%.

There were no side effects in the group treated with N. sativa oil lotion 10%.

The authors attributed the results to the antimicrobial, immunomodulatory and anti-inflammatory effects of N. sativa oil." REF - 'Propionibacterium acnes and chronic diseases'

In a review study conducted in 2015, "Only articles substantiated by appropriate scientific methodology were reviewed and included. The following are categories of the studies reviewed: antimicrobial, antiviral, antifungal, antiparasitic, wound healing, psoriasis, acne vulgaris, vitiligo, skin cancer, percutaneous absorption, cosmetic application and cutaneous side effects." Plenty of evidence was found for skin benefits of black cumin oil. In fact, the oldest scientific report on the benefits of black seed oil on human health in this review dated back to 1965. Specifically, black cumin had effects on gram-positive microorganisms, including Staph aureus. This review also found evidence for black seed oil's pharmacological activities, including antibacterial, antiviral, anti-fungal, ACNE, skin cancers, - REF - 'Dermatological effects of Nigella sativa'

Eczema
Eczema, otherwise known as atopic dermatitis, is a recurring, non-infectious, inflammatory skin condition that is commonly experienced by people with a family history of an atopic disorder, including asthma and hay fever.

In 2013, in a head-to-head study of 60 people comparing a pharmaceutical product to black cumin on hand eczema, it was found, "It seems that Nigella might have the same efficacy as Betamethasone in improvement of life quality and decreasing severity of hand eczema." - REF - 'Comparison of therapeutic effect of topical Nigella with Betamethasone and Eucerin in hand eczema'

References
'Effect of Nigella sativa (the black seed) on immunity.' In: Proceedings of the Fourth International Conference on

Islamic Medicine, 4 November, Kuwait, pp. 344–348.

'Propionibacterium acnes and chronic diseases' available from: https://www.ncbi.nlm.nih.gov/books/NBK83685/ [as accessed Jan 26, 2018].

'Propionibacterium Infections' available from: http://emedicine.medscape.com/article/226337-overview? [as accessed Jan 26, 2018].

'Dermatological effects of Nigella sativa' https://www.researchgate.net/publication/276152439 (as accessed 26 Jan 2018).

'Comparison of therapeutic effect of topical Nigella with Betamethasone and Eucerin in hand eczema' - https://www.ncbi.nlm.nih.gov/pubmed/23198836 (as accessed 5 June 2018).

Acne and Eczema

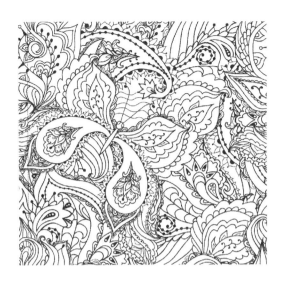

Chapter 2 - AIDS

AIDS has always been 'sold' to us as incurable, but there are a few research studies that suggest that's not true. In Africa, AIDS is a huge problem so it makes sense that the bulk of the black seed oil research in regards to this condition is to be found right there in Africa.

What is AIDS?
I'm well aware that there is a ton of controversy surrounding AIDS, including what it actually is and where it came from. There are a couple of theories, but for the sake of preserving my own health, I'm going to insert the government approved explanation,
"Acquired. This condition is acquired, meaning that a person becomes infected with it.

I - Immuno. HIV affects a person's immune system, the part of the body that fights off germs such as bacteria or viruses.

D - Deficiency. The immune system becomes deficient and does not work properly.

S - Syndrome. A person with AIDS may experience other diseases and infections because of a weakened immune system." REF - 'What is AIDS?' https://www.hiv.va.gov/patient/basics/what-is-AIDS.asp (as accessed 22 June 2018).

The Research

The Journal of Immunity Vol 12, No 4, Winter Ed. 2014/15 apparently holds the research paper from the very first patient that seroconverted after using a regimen of black seed oil. Interestingly, when I search for that on the National Center for Biotechnology Information (NCBI), every single volume of the African Journal of Traditional, Complementary, and Alternative Medicines is available except this one. Never mind, I tracked it down and now there are six patients that have been cured of AIDS with the powerful black seed. Dr Onifade has been the lead author of 4 published studies on black seed and AIDS and is finding astounding results.

On a dosage of 10mls daily for 6 months, the first documented case of curing AIDS with black seed is holding firm on the sero-reconversion after 24 months. It sure looks a lot like a cure! "This case report reflects the fact that there are possible therapeutic agents in Nigella sativa that may effectively control HIV infection." REF - '5-Month Herbal Therapy and Complete Sero-Reversion with Recovery in an Adult HIV/AIDS Patient'

Here is another of Dr Onifade's research papers on AIDS in 6 patients. This time, he used a product called 'α-Zam' which is a mix of black seed and honey. "The symptoms and signs associated with HIV infection disappeared within 20 days of commencement of herbal therapy." These 6 patients were followed up with on a daily basis for 4 months and Dr Onifade gets the last word on this, "This study concluded that the herbal remedy (α-Zam) is effective in the treatment of HIV infection based on a significant improvement in both the clinical features and laboratory results of HIV infection." REF - 'Effectiveness of a herbal remedy in six HIV patients in Nigeria'

Dr Onifade strikes again with a documented case of a 27-year-old woman that sero-reconverted in a year by taking the Nigella sativa and honey therapy (60: 40 respectively) of 10mls 3 times daily. This woman presented at an antenatal clinic in 2004 and went on to have 3 children in total, none of which contracted AIDS. This research paper was published in 2015, a full 10 years after the year of treatment with this wonder substance! REF - 'Seronegative conversion of an HIV positive subject treated with Nigella sativa and honey'

References

'What is AIDS?'
https://www.hiv.va.gov/patient/basics/what-is-AIDS.asp (as accessed 22 June 2018).

'5-Month Herbal Therapy and Complete Sero-Reversion with Recovery in an Adult HIV/AIDS Patient'
https://www.omicsonline.org/scientific-reports/1948-5964-SR124.pdf (as accessed 22 June 2018).

'Effectiveness of a herbal remedy in six HIV patients in Nigeria'
https://www.researchgate.net/publication/257321875

'Seronegative conversion of an HIV positive subject treated with Nigella sativa and honey'
https://www.researchgate.net/publication/281193905 (as accessed 22 June 2018).

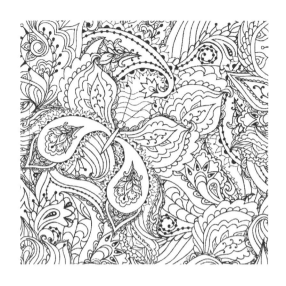

Chapter 3 - Allergies

The estimate is that 1 in 5 people in the Western world has at least 1 allergy. That's a lot of us affected. The reasons why are not for discussion here, just the possible solution. Pharmaceutical companies are happy to sell you steroid nasal sprays, antihistamines and decongestants, but they don't treat the underlying cause of the allergy, only the symptoms.

What are Allergies?
When your immune system reacts to something that is normally harmless, you have an allergy. From a runny nose and watering eyes, all the way through to anaphylactic shock and death is what can result from allergies. Wouldn't it be great if we had a cheap and effective method at our

disposal to stop the immune system from overreacting?

The Research

We have known about black seed's ability as an anti-histamine from as far back as 1970 when Marozzi et al. found significant antihistamine effects. "An inhaled Thymoquinone aerosol dose-dependently protected guinea pigs against histamine-stimulated bronchospasm in the range of 2.5–10 mg/kg"

There is more research on black seed being an antihistamine but it's mainly been performed in relation to asthma. I did, however, find a bunch of patents for allergy products that include black seed as a constituent for alleviating symptoms.

In a study on rabbits, the researchers found "The findings of a present study show that oral pre-treatment with Nigella sativa essential oil attenuates the ocular allergic response in rabbits that is produced by compound 48/80. Conclusion: Our findings suggest that Nigella sativa essential oil has mast cells stabilizing property" REF - 'Preventive Effect of Nigella Sativa Essential Oil on Signs of Ocular Allergy Induced by Compound 48/80 in Rabbits'

Another study was focused on guinea pigs' trachea and the researchers think that black seed has a blocking effect on the muscarinic receptors. REF - 'Inhibitory Effect of Nigella sativa on Histamine Receptors of Isolated Guinea Pig Tracheal Chains'

In Turkey in 2010, there was a study done on 24 people that were sensitive to house dust mites with allergic rhinitis that were also receiving specific immunotherapy. These people were compared against a control group of 8 healthy people. During this study, it was discovered that "The CD8 counts of patients receiving specific immunotherapy plus N. sativa seed supplementation significantly increased compared to patients receiving only specific immunotherapy. PMN functions of healthy volunteers significantly increased after N. sativa seed supplementation compared to baseline." REF - 'Potential adjuvant effects of Nigella sativa seeds to improve specific immunotherapy in allergic rhinitis patients'

References

https://www.sciencedirect.com/topics/medicine-and-dentistry/Thymoquinone

'Preventive Effect of Nigella Sativa Essential Oil on Signs of Ocular Allergy Induced by Compound 48/80 in Rabbits' - Pakistan Journal of Medical & Health Sciences VOL. 6 NO. 2 APR-JUN 2012

'Inhibitory Effect of Nigella sativa on Histamine Receptors of Isolated Guinea Pig Tracheal Chains' Pharmaceutical Biology 2002, Vol. 40, No. 8, pp.596-602

'Potential adjuvant effects of Nigella sativa seeds to improve specific immunotherapy in allergic rhinitis patients' https://www.ncbi.nlm.nih.gov/pubmed/20357504 (as accessed 23 June 2018).

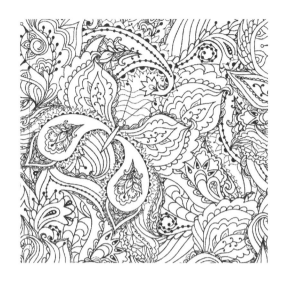

Chapter 4 – Autism

There isn't a lot of scientific research available on this subject, after all, you can't patent Nature, so when big pharma does their research on plants, it isn't published generally. When Nature is investigated by pharma, it's for the purpose of adding chemicals to it for a patent. With no compulsion to ever publish any scientific research, do you think they would release research that touts the benefits of Nature alone?

What is Autism?
Autism is a behavioural disorder associated with neurological impairment. In the world of scientific research, it is a relatively young subject of study, and as such, doesn't

have a great deal of studies available to reference. This means we have to cast the research net a little wider.

There is no blood test for autism but they are working on it. And as yet, none of the mainstream allopathic doctors and researchers have found a cure. However, many parents of autistic children are finding some relief from autism symptoms as attested to by many anecdotes to be found wherever there is an autism chat going on. Black seed is one of the substances that those parents are talking about.

In my research, I found some VERY encouraging anecdotal stories about black seed oil helping to reduce the symptoms of autistic children. While I cannot quote the parents' comments here, I can help you find them online.

I now use duckduckgo.com as my search engine because they say they don't record your searches, but use whichever you prefer and type in searches like 'autism relief forum' or 'forum natural remedy autism' and you will start to see what others are saying. In fact, I did do a couple of those searches and found autismforums.com, autismweb.com/forum, topix.com/forum/health/autism and dealwithautism.com/forum.

The Research
There is some research going on with autism (listed below) but not nearly enough. This is where anecdotes come in to fill the gap. For thousands of years of anecdotal healing and

learning, people are still helping people by sharing their stories with each other. Healing methods that have stood the test of time are being retold, over and over, down the line of many generations. Just because science hasn't bothered to catch up doesn't mean you or anyone else should miss out on the chance to heal. Remember what Dr Wakefield says, *"The anecdote is where medicine begins."*

The Muslim community is very reliant on the amazing healing power of black seed oil, and this is because it's mentioned in the herbs section of the Qu-ran as "The remedy for all ailments except death"

When I couldn't find any direct research linking autism to black cumin, I went looking for any brain-related studies. I found a few...

In a study called 'Feeding of Nigella sativa during neonatal and juvenile growth improves learning and memory of rats', it was found that...
"Neurodevelopmental alterations in the frontal/prefrontal cortex, striatum, and hippocampus, which are heavily involved in cognition, memory, emotion, and learning, are likely involved in the etiology of neuropsychiatric disorders like autism, substance use disorders, schizophrenia, Parkinson's disease, and Alzheimer's disease."- REF - 'Feeding of Nigella sativa during neonatal and juvenile growth improves learning and memory of rats'

In a review study, it has been noted that "...recently emerging studies conducted with animal models suggest that Thymoquinone – bearing a very simple molecular structure – significantly crosses the blood-brain barrier and exerts neuromodulatory activities. Indeed, in animal studies, the following actions of Thymoquinone were demonstrated;

1 – Protection against ischemic brain damage.
2 – Reduction of epileptic seizures and associated cerebral oxidative injury.
3 – Reduction of morphine tolerance and associated oxidative brain damage.
4 – Anxiolytic effects and reduction of immobility stress-associated cerebral oxidative injury.
5 – Reduction of diabetes-induced cerebral oxidative stress.
6 – Reduction of cerebral oxidative injuries induced by noxious exposures including toluene, lead and ionizing radiation." - REF - 'Thymoquinone: An edible redox-active quinone for the pharmacotherapy of neurodegenerative conditions and glial brain tumours. A short review'

"Substantial in vitro data suggest that Thymoquinone may be beneficial in treatment of glial tumours. However, there is no clinical study investigating its antitumor effects. In fact, Thymoquinone suppresses growth and invasion, and induces apoptosis of glial tumour cells via degrading tubulins and inhibiting 20S proteasome, telomerase, autophagy, FAK and metalloproteinases. A simple and easily available agent may be a promising adjunctive treatment option in neurological and neurosurgical practice."- REF - 'Feeding of Nigella sativa during neonatal and juvenile growth improves learning and memory of rats'

Then There's Encephalomyelitis

Another school of thought is that autism is an inflammation of the brain, a form of encephalomyelitis. If that's what we are looking at here, then the quote below is very encouraging for the autism affected because the black seed appears to be rebuilding the myelin sheath.

"The ultrastructural examination of the "EAE" group revealed partial to complete demyelination in the medulla (Figure 4) in addition to thin and marked myelin destruction with severe myelinolysis of nerve fibres in the cerebellum (Figure 5). These changes were alleviated in N. sativa treated and protected groups. TEM micrographs of the brain areas of "EAE + N. sativa" group showed partial to complete remyelination in the medulla besides complete remyelination of most nerve fibres in the cerebellum with well-developed myelin sheath. In addition, most of the myelinated fibres in the "N. sativa + EAE" group were in a state of remyelination in the cerebellum and medulla." REF - 'Nigella sativa amliorates inflammation and demyelination in the experimental autoimmune encephalomyelitis-induced Wistar rats'

What Did All That Have to Do with Autism?

This could be great news for those with autism, as a possible avenue to pursue, seeing as they say they don't know what causes it yet but it is some sort of dysfunction of the brain and the gut has been heavily implicated too.

References

'Alternative therapies in health and medicine' https://www.researchgate.net/publication/23930234 (as accessed 3 Feb 2018).

'Thymoquinone: An edible redox-active quinone for the pharmacotherapy of neurodegenerative conditions and glial brain tumours. A short review' https://www.sciencedirect.com/science/article/pii/S07533322 16307302 (as accessed 4 Feb 2018).

'Feeding of Nigella sativa during neonatal and juvenile growth improves learning and memory of rats' https://www.sciencedirect.com/science/article/pii/S22254110 14000534 (as accessed 4 Feb 2018).

'Indian Medicinal Plants: A Compendium of 500 Species' - Warrier PK, Nambiar VPK, Ramankutty. Chennai: Orient Longman Pvt Ltd; 2004

Yarnell E, Abascal K. - 'Nigella sativa: holy herb of the Middle East'

'The Uncomfortable Truth About Dr Wakefield And Why

Your Story of Vaccine Injury Is "Essential" – 6319 Stories and Counting!'
https://www.naturalnewsblogs.com/uncomfortable-truth-dr-wakefield-story-vaccine-injury-essential-6319-stories-counting/ (as accessed 3 Feb 2018).

https://myautisticmuslimchild.wordpress.com/about/

'Nigella sativa amliorates inflammation and demyelination in the experimental autoimmune encephalomyelitis-induced Wistar rats' -
https://www.ncbi.nlm.nih.gov/pmc/articles/PMC4525838/ (as accessed 10 June 2018).

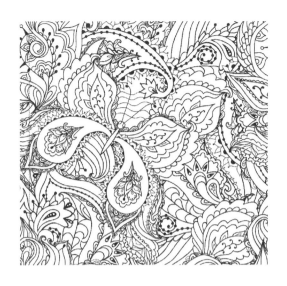

Chapter 5 – Cancer

"Thymoquinone modulates nine of the ten hallmarks of cancer." - REF - "Thymoquinone: fifty years of success in the battle against cancer models'

There are many research studies that show great results for black seed oil treatments related to its cancer-killing and anti-inflammatory properties.

What is Cancer?
Well, of course, that depends on what type of cancer we are talking about. In its most basic explanation, cancer is cells gone wrong. The cause of which is most often not discovered. There are benign cancers and malignant cancers. It's the latter you have to worry about.

The Research

There have been many studies that have shown the effects of Nigella sativa on many different cancers and I will quote just a few of them here. The full list of research studies that I found is included at the end of this chapter. The list is long!

Even doctors are now urging more research into Thymoquinone (TQ), the main constituent in black seed oil, for adjuvants to pharmaceutical cancer treatments – REF - 'Thymoquinone as a Potential Adjuvant Therapy for Cancer Treatment: Evidence from Preclinical Studies.'

What the scientists are looking to discover are the exact signalling pathways that help black cumin seed oil play such a big role in killing cancer.

Many Pathways to Healing

"The anti-cancer effects of Thymoquinone are mediated through different modes of action, including anti-proliferation, apoptosis induction, cell cycle arrest, ROS generation and anti-metastasis/anti-angiogenesis. In addition, this quinone was found to exhibit anti-cancer activity through the modulation of multiple molecular targets, including p53, p73, PTEN, STAT3, PPAR-γ, activation of caspases and generation of ROS.

Thymoquinone is an active ingredient isolated from Nigella sativa and has been investigated for its antioxidant, anti-inflammatory and anti-cancer activities in both vitro and vivo models since its first extraction in the 1960s.

Its antioxidant/anti-inflammatory effect has been reported in various disease models, including encephalomyelitis, diabetes, asthma and carcinogenesis.

In addition, Thymoquinone could act as a free radical and superoxide radical scavenger, as well as preserving the activity of various antioxidant enzymes such as catalase, glutathione peroxidase and glutathione-S-transferase." REF - 'Thymoquinone: Potential cure for inflammatory disorders and cancer'

More Amazing Cancer Research with Black Seed Oil
"As non-invasive lesions progress to malignancy, the precursor period provides a window for cancer therapies that can interfere with neoplastic progression. Thymoquinone (TQ), a major bioactive component of essential oil from Nigella sativa's seeds, has demonstrated antineoplastic activities in multiple cancers" REF - 'Molecular Analysis of Precursor Lesions in Familial Pancreatic Cancer'

"A cell study conducted at the International Immuno – Biology Research Laboratory in South Carolina showed that when incubated with Nigella extract, cancer cells were unable to produce fibroblast growth factor and the protein collagenase, both are necessary for blood-vessel growth into the tumour. Without a blood supply, a tumour cannot grow." REF - 'Hormonal Contents of Two Types of Black Seed (Nigella sativa) Oil: Comparative Study'

"Thymoquinone blocked angiogenesis in vitro and in vivo, prevented tumour angiogenesis in a xenograft human prostate cancer (PC3) model in mouse, and inhibited human prostate tumour growth at low dosage with almost no chemotoxic side effects. Overall, our results indicate that Thymoquinone inhibits tumour angiogenesis and tumour growth and could be used as a potential drug candidate for cancer therapy." REF - 'Thymoquinone inhibits tumour angiogenesis and tumour growth through suppressing AKT and extracellular signal-regulated kinase signalling pathways'

"In fact, Thymoquinone suppresses growth and invasion, and induces apoptosis of glial tumour cells via degrading tubulins and inhibiting 20S proteasome, telomerase, autophagy, FAK and metalloproteinases. A simple and easily available agent may be a promising adjunctive treatment option in neurological and neurosurgical practice." REF - 'Thymoquinone: An edible redox-active quinone for the pharmacotherapy of neurodegenerative conditions and glial brain tumours. A short review'
"TQ was found to increase sub-G1 accumulation and annexin-V positive staining, indicating apoptotic induction." REF - 'Anticancer activity of Thymoquinone in breast cancer cells: Possible involvement of PPAR-γ pathway'

"Thymoquinone from Nigella sativa was more potent than cisplatin in eliminating of SiHa cells via apoptosis with down-regulation of Bcl-2 protein." REF - 'Thymoquinone from Nigella sativa was more potent than cisplatin in eliminating of SiHa cells via apoptosis with down-regulation of Bcl-2 protein'

In the International Journal of Oncology, we find a study that tells us "Thymoquinone extracted from black seed triggers apoptotic cell death in human colorectal cancer cells via a p53-dependent mechanism." They also had this to say, "These results indicate that TQ is antineoplastic and pro-apoptotic against colon cancer cell line HCT116. The apoptotic effects of TQ are modulated by Bcl-2 protein and are linked to and dependent on p53. Our data support the potential for using the agent TQ for the treatment of colon cancer."

From the same study, "Thymoquinone extracted from black seed triggers apoptotic cell death in human colorectal cancer cells via a p53-dependent mechanism."

Still from the same study, "These results indicate that TQ is antineoplastic and pro-apoptotic against colon cancer cell line HCT116. The apoptotic effects of TQ are modulated by Bcl-2 protein and are linked to and dependent on p53. Our data support the potential for using the agent TQ for the treatment of colon cancer." Meaning the black seed oil is killing cancer cells! REF - 'Thymoquinone extracted from black seed triggers apoptotic cell death in human colorectal cancer cells via a p53-dependent mechanism'

From a 2003 study, we find that "Thymoquinone inhibits autophagy and induces cathepsin-mediated, caspase-independent cell death in glioblastoma cells." More cancer cell killing evidence. REF - 'Thymoquinone Inhibits Autophagy and Induces Cathepsin-Mediated, Caspase-Independent Cell Death in Glioblastoma Cells'

From another study in 2003, the good news for epilepsy sufferers is that "These findings demonstrate that the volatile oil of N. sativa has the ability to inhibit colon carcinogenesis of rats in the post-initiation stage, with no evident adverse side effects, and that the inhibition may be associated, in part, with suppression of cell proliferation in the colonic mucosa" REF - 'Chemopreventive potential of volatile oil from black cumin (Nigella sativa L.) seeds against rat colon carcinogenesis'

The very best research on the effect of black cumin on cancers was conducted through a review of research papers in 2011. In this study, the role of black cumin as an anti-cancer agent is explained, thus, "Many active ingredients have been found in the seeds of N. sativa. The seeds contain both fixed and essential oils, proteins, alkaloids and saponin described the quantification of four pharmacologically important components: Thymoquinone (TQ), Dithymoquinone (DTQ), Thymohydroquinone (THQ), and thymol (THY), in the oil of N. sativa seed by HPLC. Much of the biological activities of the seeds have been shown to be due to Thymoquinone, the major component of the essential oil, which is also present in the fixed oil"

In a review study, the researchers have offered up 57 reviewed research papers on this subject and found black cumin to be effective against these cancers:

- Blood cancer - El-Mahdy et al. (2005), Effenberger et al. (2010), Swamy and Huat (2003)
- Breast cancer - Farah and Begum (2003), (El-Aziz et al., 2005), Effenberger et al. (2010)
- Colon cancer - Gali-Muhtasib et al. (2004), Salim and Fukushima (2003), Norwood et al. (2006)
- Pancreatic cancer - Chehl et al. (2009), Banerjee et al., (2009), Torres et al. (2010)
- Hepatic cancer - Thabrew et al. (2005), Nagi and Almakki (2009)
- Lung cancer - Swamy and Huat (2003), Mabrouk et al. (2002)
- Leukemia - El-Mahdy et al. (2005)
- Skin cancer - Salomi et al. (1991)
- Fibrosarcoma - Badary and Gamal (2001)
- Renal cancer - Khan and Sultana (2005)
- Prostate cancer - Kaseb et al. (2007), Yi et al. (2008)
- Cervical cancer - Shafi et al. (2009), Effenberger et al. (2010)
REF - 'Anticancer Activities of Nigella Sativa (Black Cumin)'

Already Getting Chemotherapy?

You might want to have a look at the study from 2010 that tested the effectiveness of protection afforded by black cumin against the toxicity of the drug cyclophosphamide. The researchers stated, "These results suggest that administration of NSO or TQ can lower CTX-induced toxicity as shown by an up-regulation of antioxidant mechanisms, indicating a potential clinical application for these agents to minimize the toxic effects of treatment with anticancer drugs." REF - 'Protective effects of Nigella sativa oil and Thymoquinone against toxicity induced by the anticancer drug cyclophosphamide'

Protection Against Radiotherapy

In 2009 in a study of 60 rats, it was found that "Our results strongly recommend Nigella sativa oil as a promising natural radioprotective agent against immunosuppressive and oxidative effects of ionizing radiation." REF - 'Radioprotective effects of black seed (Nigella sativa) oil against hemopoietic damage and immunosuppression in gamma-irradiated rats'

As you can see, there is a LOT of potential healing to be had with the little black cumin seed, even on cancers. There is so much research available that it begs the question, "Why aren't cancer patients routinely treated with black cumin seed oil?"

References

'Modulation of apoptosis in human hepatocellular carcinoma (HepG2 cells) by a standardized herbal decoction of Nigella sativa seeds, Hemidesmus indicus roots and Smilax glabra rhizomes with anti- hepatocarcinogenic effects.' https://www.ncbi.nlm.nih.gov/pubmed/22458551 (as accessed 31 Jan 2018).

'Protective effects of Nigella sativa oil and Thymoquinone against toxicity induced by the anticancer drug cyclophosphamide' https://www.ncbi.nlm.nih.gov/pubmed/20373678 (as accessed 31 Jan 2018).

'Anticancer Activities of Nigella Sativa (Black Cumin)' https://www.ncbi.nlm.nih.gov/pmc/articles/PMC3252704/ (as accessed 31 Jan 2018).

Thymoquinone as a Potential Adjuvant Therapy for Cancer Treatment: Evidence from Preclinical Studies.' https://www.ncbi.nlm.nih.gov/pubmed/28659794 (as accessed 4 Feb 2018).

'Thymoquinone: fifty years of success in the battle against cancer models' https://www.sciencedirect.com/science/article/pii/S13596446 13002882 (as accessed 31 Jan 2018).

'Molecular Analysis of Precursor Lesions in Familial

Pancreatic Cancer'
https://www.researchgate.net/publication/235393451 (as
accessed 4 Feb 2018).

'Hormonal Contents of Two Types of Black Seed (Nigella
sativa) Oil: Comparative Study'
https://www.iasj.net/iasj?func=fulltext&aId=42676 (as
accessed 4 Feb 2018).

'Thymoquinone inhibits tumour angiogenesis and tumour
growth through suppressing AKT and extracellular signal-
regulated kinase signalling pathways'
https://www.ncbi.nlm.nih.gov/pubmed/18644991 (as
accessed 4 Feb 2018).

Thymoquinone: An edible redox-active quinone for the
pharmacotherapy of neurodegenerative conditions and glial
brain tumours. A short review'
https://www.sciencedirect.com/science/article/pii/S07533322
16307302 (as accessed 4 Feb 2018).

'Anticancer activity of Thymoquinone in breast cancer cells:
Possible involvement of PPAR-γ pathway'
https://www.sciencedirect.com/science/article/pii/S00062952
11003637 (as accessed 4 Feb 2018).

Thymoquinone from Nigella sativa was more potent than
cisplatin in eliminating of SiHa cells via apoptosis with
down-regulation of Bcl-2 protein'

https://www.sciencedirect.com/science/article/pii/S08872333 11001366 (as accessed 4 Feb 2018).

'Thymoquinone extracted from black seed triggers apoptotic cell death in human colorectal cancer cells via a p53-dependent mechanism'
https://www.researchgate.net/publication/8338395 (as accessed 4 Feb 2018).

Thymoquinone Inhibits Autophagy and Induces Cathepsin-Mediated, Caspase-Independent Cell Death in Glioblastoma Cells'
http://journals.plos.org/plosone/article?id=10.1371/journal.pone.0072882 (as accessed 4 Feb 2018).

'Chemopreventive potential of volatile oil from black cumin (Nigella sativa L.) seeds against rat colon carcinogenesis'

http://www.tandfonline.com/doi/abs/10.1207/S15327914NC4 502_09 (as accessed 4 Feb 2018).

'Radioprotective effects of black seed (Nigella sativa) oil against hemopoietic damage and immunosuppression in gamma-irradiated rats'
http://www.tandfonline.com/doi/full/10.3109/0892397090330 7552 (as accessed 4 Feb 2018).

More Research!
The list of research into black cumin against cancer is vast.

When you search PubMed online for 'Thymoquinone and cancer', you get 271 results returned. When you search 'Nigella sativa and cancer', you get 201 results. Here are a few more research papers to get you started on your journey...

'Thymoquinone Promotes Pancreatic Cancer Cell Death and Reduction of Tumour Size through Combined Inhibition of Histone Deacetylation and Induction of Histone Acetylation' https://www.ncbi.nlm.nih.gov/pubmed/28105374 (as accessed 9 Feb 2018).

'Recent advances on the anti-cancer properties of Nigella sativa, a widely used food additive' https://www.ncbi.nlm.nih.gov/pmc/articles/PMC5052360/ (as accessed 9 Feb 2018).

'Thymoquinone chemosensitizes colon cancer cells through inhibition of NF-κB' https://www.ncbi.nlm.nih.gov/pubmed/27698868 (as accessed 9 Feb 2018).

'Anticancer activity of Thymoquinone in breast cancer cells: possible involvement of PPAR-γ pathway' https://www.ncbi.nlm.nih.gov/pubmed/21679698 (as accessed 9 Feb 2018).

'Cytotoxicity of Nigella sativa seed oil and extract against human lung cancer cell line' https://www.ncbi.nlm.nih.gov/pubmed/24568529 (as accessed 9 Feb 2018).

'Thymoquinone inhibits tumour angiogenesis and tumour growth through suppressing AKT and extracellular signal-regulated kinase signalling pathways' http://mct.aacrjournals.org/content/7/7/1789 (as accessed 9 Feb 2018).

'Cellular responses with Thymoquinone treatment in human breast cancer cell line MCF-7' https://www.ncbi.nlm.nih.gov/pubmed/2390012(as accessed 9 Feb 2018).

'Thymoquinone from Nigella sativa was more potent than cisplatin in eliminating of SiHa cells via apoptosis with down-regulation of Bcl-2 protein' https://www.ncbi.nlm.nih.gov/pubmed/21609759 (as accessed 9 Feb 2018).

'A comparison of 5-fluorouracil and natural chemotherapeutic agents, EGCG and Thymoquinone, delivered by sustained drug delivery on colon cancer cells' https://www.ncbi.nlm.nih.gov/pubmed/17487093 (as accessed 9 Feb 2018).

'In vitro inhibition of growth and induction of apoptosis in cancer cell lines by Thymoquinone' https://www.ncbi.nlm.nih.gov/pubmed/12469192 (as

accessed 9 Feb 2018).

'Thymoquinone extracted from black seed triggers apoptotic cell death in human colorectal cancer cells via a p53-dependent mechanism' https://www.ncbi.nlm.nih.gov/pubmed/15375533 (as accessed 9 Feb 2018).

'Thymoquinone and cisplatin as a therapeutic combination in lung cancer: In vitro and in vivo' https://www.ncbi.nlm.nih.gov/pubmed/20594324 (as accessed 9 Feb 2018).

'Effect of Thymoquinone on P53 Gene Expression and Consequence Apoptosis in Breast Cancer Cell Line' https://www.ncbi.nlm.nih.gov/pmc/articles/PMC4837800/ (as accessed 9 Feb 2018).

'Thymoquinone inhibits autophagy and induces cathepsin-mediated, caspase-independent cell death in glioblastoma cells' https://www.ncbi.nlm.nih.gov/pubmed/24039814 (as accessed 9 Feb 2018).

'Antitumor and anti-angiogenesis effects of Thymoquinone on osteosarcoma through the NF-κB pathway' https://www.ncbi.nlm.nih.gov/pubmed/23232982 (as accessed 9 Feb 2018).

'Thymoquinone: potential cure for inflammatory disorders and cancer' https://www.ncbi.nlm.nih.gov/pubmed/22005518 (as accessed 9 Feb 2018).

'Observations on the Biological Effects of Black Cumin Seed (Nigella sativa) and Green Tea (Camellia sinensis)' http://idosi.org/gv/gv2(4)08/9.pdf (as accessed 9 Feb 2018). 'Thymoquinone: a promising anti-cancer drug from natural sources' https://www.ncbi.nlm.nih.gov/pubmed/16314136 (as accessed 9 Feb 2018).

'Anti-inflammatory effects of the Nigella sativa seed extract, Thymoquinone, in pancreatic cancer cells' https://www.ncbi.nlm.nih.gov/pubmed/19768141 (as accessed 9 Feb 2018).

'Methanolic extract of Nigella sativa seed inhibits SiHa human cervical cancer cell proliferation through apoptosis' https://www.ncbi.nlm.nih.gov/pubmed/23513732 (as accessed 9 Feb 2018).

'Thymoquinone from Nigella sativa was more potent than cisplatin in eliminating of SiHa cells via apoptosis with down-regulation of Bcl-2 protein' https://www.ncbi.nlm.nih.gov/pubmed/21609759 (as accessed 9 Feb 2018).

'Chemopreventive potential of volatile oil from black cumin (Nigella sativa L.) seeds against rat colon carcinogenesis' https://www.ncbi.nlm.nih.gov/pubmed/12881014 (as accessed 9 Feb 2018).

Cancer

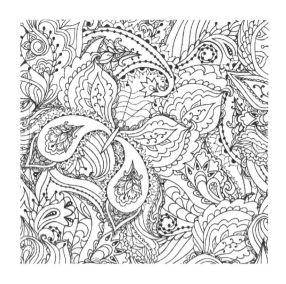

Chapter 6 – Candida

Here is yet another mass of studies that have been conducted showing black seed's ability to fight imbalance in the body.

What is Candida?
An online medical dictionary tells us, "...a genus of yeast-like fungi that are commonly part of the normal flora of the mouth, skin, intestinal tract, and vagina, but can cause a variety of infections. C. albicans is the usual pathogen in humans." REF – Thefreedictionary.com

Candida being the main culprit for vaginal thrush, which all us women will be afflicted with at one time or another, can be caused by damn near anything. Any natural treatment for this is highly prized and, yes, black cumin can help with this problem. BUT, do NOT ever put undiluted black seed oil on or in your vagina! OWW! Ingestion is a far better route as this stuff is spicy and I can imagine it would burn the heck out of any sensitive bits.

When we take antibiotics/antibacterials for long enough, candida inevitably shows up and can be more in its pathogenic fungal form. Thus creating a whole different set of problems. If you are prone to candida, try to stay away from antibiotics and antibacterial products, please!

The Research

I found a fair bit of research when it comes to getting rid of candida with black seed, for instance, "The research shows treatment with natural products in a good light as an alternative for treating fungal infections. The authors envisage Nigella sativa extract enhancing the effect of conventional therapy" REF - 'An alternative treatment for Candida infections with Nigella sativa extracts'

"The extract (black cumin) successfully eradicated a non-fatal subcutaneous staphylococcal infection in mice when injected at the site of infection." REF - 'Studies on the antimicrobial activity of Nigella sativa seed (black cumin)'

"These results indicate that the aqueous extract of Nigella sativa seeds exhibits an inhibitory effect against candidiasis and this study validates the traditional use of the plant in fungal infections" – REF - 'The in vivo antifungal activity of the aqueous extract from Nigella sativa seeds'

Scientific Review

"The ether extract of N. sativa was reported to inhibit the growth of Candida yeasts in several organs in experimental animal infections." REF - 'Dermatological effects of Nigella sativa'

References

https://medical-dictionary.thefreedictionary.com/Candida

'An alternative treatment for Candida infections with Nigella sativa extracts'
https://www.researchgate.net/publication/273646893 (as accessed 4 Feb 2018).

'Studies on the antimicrobial activity of Nigella sativa seed (black cumin)'
https://www.sciencedirect.com/science/article/pii/037887419 190047H (as accessed 23 June 2018).

'The in vivo antifungal activity of the aqueous extract from Nigella sativa seeds'
https://www.ncbi.nlm.nih.gov/pubmed/12601685 (as accessed 4 Feb 2018).

'Dermatological effects of Nigella sativa'
https://www.sciencedirect.com/science/article/pii/S23522410 15000286 (as accessed 4 Feb 2018).

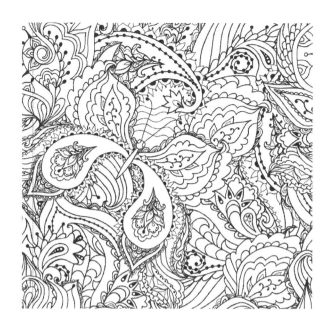

Chapter 7 – Constipation

There are so many healing abilities attributed to the humble black seed oil, constipation relief being one of them. Most oils will help constipation by taking a tablespoon on a regular basis, and black seed is no different.

What is Constipation?
This is such a common complaint, so we all know that constipation means you can't poo.

The Research
Not a lot of research has been done on this aspect of the black cumin seed, in fact, I couldn't find any.

All oils, when taken internally, help to lubricate and soften stools for ease of elimination.

For some relief from constipation, you should really give the humble black cumin seed oil a try.

References

My own experience with black seed oil has been that it does indeed aid with 'slide-and-deliver' when it was needed.

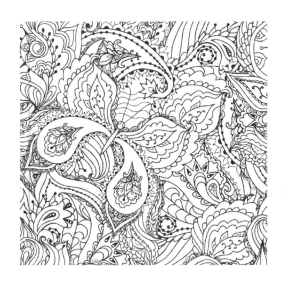

Chapter 8 – Contraindications and Interactions

There are many pharmaceutical drugs that may interfere with the black seed oil pharmacological pathways to healing due to the many actions it can perform. Pharmaceuticals can affect black seed oil's intestinal availability and pharmacological effect. And, vice versa, of course.

What are Contraindications and Interactions?
When a substance interferes with the correct function of another, it's called a contraindication. When a substance changes the way another substance (usually a pharmaceutical drug) works, it's called an interaction. Neither of which you want to go on inside your body.

Contraindications and Interactions

The Research

Black seed oil has been known to increase the effectiveness of analgesics and Cox-2 inhibitors. As always, you should check with your health care provider, especially if you are on prescription medications.

In one study, "It also showed synergistic effect with streptomycin and gentamycin and additive effect with spectinomycin, erythromycin, tobramycin, doxycycline, chloramphenicol, nalidixic acid, ampicillin, lincomycin and co-trimoxazole and successfully eradicated a non-fatal subcutaneous staphylococcal infection induced experimentally in mice when injected at the site of infection (Hanafi and Hatem, 1991)." REF - 'Dermatological effects of Nigella sativa'

LIKELY SAFE: When used orally in amounts found in foods.

POSSIBLY SAFE: When black seed oil or black seed extract is used in medicinal amounts, short-term.

CHILDREN POSSIBLY SAFE: When black seed oil is used orally in recommended amounts, short-term.

USE IN PREGNANCY LIKELY UNSAFE

When used orally in amounts exceeding those found in food, black seed may decrease or inhibit uterine contractions and may have contraceptive action.

Amoxicillin

There was a study done in 2012 to investigate the effect on the bioavailability of amoxicillin in rats when co-administered with black cumin. This study concluded that, yes, taking black cumin at the same time as amoxicillin increased intestinal absorption rates. - REF - 'Bioavailability enhancement studies of amoxicillin with Nigella.'

Blood Clotting Agents

Black seed can slow blood clotting. Taking black seed along with medications that also slow blood clotting might increase the chances of bruising and bleeding.

Decrease Blood Pressure

Black seed might decrease blood pressure in some people. Taking black seed along with medications used for lowering high blood pressure might cause your blood pressure to go too low.

Do not take black seed if you are taking medications for high blood pressure.

Stop using black seed at least two weeks before a scheduled surgery.

Immune Depressive Drugs

Black seed oil acts as an immuno-modulator on the immune system. By its action of boosting the immune system, black seed might decrease the effectiveness of immunosuppressant medications that decrease immune system response. REF –

'Black Seed'

Pregnancy and Breast Feeding

Black seed seems to be safe in food amounts during pregnancy. But taking larger medicinal amounts is LIKELY UNSAFE. Black seed can slow down or stop the uterus from contracting.

Not much is known about the safety of using black seed during breastfeeding. Stay on the safe side and avoid the use of it altogether.

Sleepiness

Black seed might cause sleepiness and/or drowsiness. Using black seed along with sedative medications might make you too sleepy.

Take it Easy

Look. you are going to LOVE black cumin seed oil, BUT, like any new product, start slowly and build up to regular usage. Some people find that they are skin allergic to black seed oil. Try a couple of drops on your skin to check your sensitivity. Then, over the course of a few days, take a few drops per day. If you don't have any negative reaction, then you should be safe to start dosing. But, as always, check with your health care provider first.

References

'A review on therapeutic potential of Nigella sativa: A

miracle herb'
https://www.ncbi.nlm.nih.gov/pmc/articles/PMC3642442/ (as
accessed 2 Feb 2018).

'Bioavailability enhancement studies of amoxicillin with
Nigella' https://www.ncbi.nlm.nih.gov/pubmed/22664507/
(as accessed 2 Feb 2018).

'Black Seed' http://www.emedicinehealth.com/black_seed-
page3/vitamins-supplements.htm#Interactions [as accessed 2
Feb 2018].

'Dermatological effects of Nigella sativa'
https://www.sciencedirect.com/science/article/pii/S23522410
15000286#b0005 [as accessed Jan 26, 2018].

Contraindications and Interactions

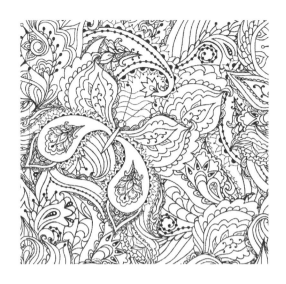

Chapter 9 – Diabetes

There is plentiful data to be found concerning the help that black cumin oil offers the diabetes sufferer. Nigella sativa is one of the few substances known to man that shows great promise in preventing both type 1 and type 2 diabetes.

What is Diabetes?

Diabetes.org.uk defines diabetes as, "... a serious life-long health condition that occurs when the amount of glucose (sugar) in the blood is too high because the body can't use it properly. If left untreated, high blood glucose levels can cause serious health complications."

The Research

Many research papers have reported that N. sativa has anti-diabetic and hypoglycemic activity. How exciting for those suffering the ill effects of diabetes and the related pharmaceutical medicines!

Like everything else, make sure you check with your health care provider if you are wanting to combine black cumin products with pharmaceuticals. Remember, the pharmacological actions of black cumin are vast. Some pharma drugs have their effect increased and other pharma drugs won't work at all when taking black cumin.

"The biochemical and ultrastructural findings suggest that N. sativa extract and Thymoquinone have therapeutic and protect against STZ-diabetes by decreasing oxidative stress, thus preserving pancreatic β-cell integrity. The hypoglycemic effect observed could be due to amelioration of β-cell ultrastructure, thus leading to increased insulin levels. Consequently, N. sativa and Thymoquinone may prove clinically useful in the treatment of diabetics and in the protection of β-cells against oxidative stress." REF - 'Effects of Nigella sativa and Thymoquinone on biochemical and subcellular changes in pancreatic β-cells of streptozotocin-induced diabetic rats.'

"These results showed that hydroalcoholic extract of NS (Nigella sativa) at low doses has hypoglycemic effect and as well as lipid profile in diabetic subjects. Nigella sativa is a potential protective natural agent against atherosclerosis, hepatoprotective and cardiovascular complication in diabetic rats." REF - 'Hypoglycemic and Hypolipidemic

Potential of Nigella sativa L. Seed Extract in Streptozotocin (STZ)-Induced Diabetic Rats'

Eventually published by the Journal of Endocrinology and Metabolism, a group of researchers from the Indian Council of Medical Research significantly found that:

"Black seed oil causes gradual partial regeneration of pancreatic beta-cells, increases the lowered serum insulin concentrations and decreases the elevated serum glucose." REF - 'Antidiabetic Properties of a Spice Plant Nigella sativa'

In fact, according to one study, "Oral administration of Thymoquinone, metformin and their nanoformulations significantly decreased blood glucose level and glycated haemoglobin; and improved the lipid profile of diabetic rats as compared to diabetic control rats. Thymoquinone-loaded NCs (containing 10, 20 and 40 mg of Thymoquinone) produced a dose-dependent antihyperglycemic effect and this effect was comparable to Thymoquinone and metformin." REF - 'Improvement of antihyperglycemic activity of Nano-Thymoquinone in rat model of type-2 diabetes'

In one study of 94 participants, it was found that "2 grams of N. sativa daily for 3 months reduced fasting blood glucose by an average of 45, 62 and 56 mg/dl at 4, 8 and 12 weeks respectively. HbAlC was reduced by 1.52% at the end of the 12 weeks of treatment ($P<0.0001$). Insulin resistance calculated by HOMA2 was reduced significantly (P<0.01), while B-cell function was increased (P<0.02) at 12 weeks of treatment." REF - 'Effect of Nigella sativa seeds on the glycemic control of patients with type 2 diabetes mellitus'

What I found most interesting in the above study was, "...Nigella sativa used in the study did not adversely affect either renal functions or hepatic functions of the diabetic patients throughout the study period." How vastly different from pharmaceuticals!

In 2009, a review of 46 animal studies looking at the efficacy of medicinal plants was undertaken. This review, 'A systematic review of the potential herbal sources of future drugs effective in oxidant-related diseases' found that "Lipid peroxidation was reduced in different clinical circumstances by Nigella sativa" and other plants."

"N. sativa reduces oxidative stress on liver cells. Positive effects have been found from the ingestion of N. sativa oil on the parameters of serum insulin, super dismutase (SOD), serum glucose and malondialdehyde (MDA) levels. This has been demonstrated in many studies (53, 56-59). Thymoquinone content of N. sativa were considered as the major constituent responsible for the antidiabetic activity of the herb. The effectiveness of N. sativa in diabetic patients is further increased if it is used along with α- lipoic acid and L-carnitine supplements" REF - 'Cardio-protective and anti-cancer therapeutic potential of Nigella sativa'

Diabetes

A clear claim to the effectiveness of black seed on diabetes; "Our data show that the antidiabetic properties of N. sativa seeds may be, at least partly, mediated by stimulated insulin release, and that the basic subfraction largely contributes to this stimulatory effect. Further phytochemical studies are underway in order to isolate the pharmacological compound(s) responsible for the insulinotropic effect of N. sativa seeds." REF - 'Nigella sativa seed extracts enhance glucose-induced insulin release from rat-isolated Langerhans islets'

Yet another study where the researchers found good evidence of protection against diabetes with black seed; "These findings suggest that NS treatment exerts a therapeutic protective effect in diabetes by decreasing oxidative stress and preserving pancreatic beta-cell integrity. Consequently, NS may be clinically useful for protecting beta-cells against oxidative stress." REF - 'Effects of Nigella sativa on oxidative stress and beta-cell damage in streptozotocin-induced diabetic rats'

I also found a study using rats that stated the "Administration of N. sativa seeds extract improved considerably, serum lipids of diabetic rats which were however not completely normal. Oxidative stress plays a role in the causation of diabetes and Antioxidants have been shown to have a role in the alleviation of diabetes" REF - Indian Journal of Experiential Biology '

Another study that I found suggests that black seed is useful for diabetic disorders; "N. sativa seed extracts exhibited significant hypoglycaemic and hypolipidaemic effects. The most important action of Nigella sativa that may be responsible for its beneficial effect in metabolic syndrome is its insulin-sensitizing action. N. sativa treatment may indicate its usefulness as a potential treatment in diabetic patients, our results suggested that hydroalcoholic extract of NS (Nigella sativa) at low doses has a beneficial effect on FBG level and ameliorative effect on regeneration of pancreatic islets and may be used as a therapeutic agent in the management of diabetes mellitus." REF - 'Hypoglycemic and Hypolipidemic Potential of Nigella sativa L. Seed Extract in Streptozotocin (STZ)-Induced Diabetic Rats'

References

'Effect of Nigella sativa seeds on the glycemic control of patients with type 2 diabetes mellitus.' https://www.ncbi.nlm.nih.gov/pubmed/21675032 (as accessed 29 Jan 2018).

'Cardio-protective and anti-cancer therapeutic potential of Nigella sativa' https://www.ncbi.nlm.nih.gov/pmc/articles/PMC4387232/ (as accessed 9 Feb 2018).

'Antidiabetic Properties of a Spice Plant Nigella sativa' - http://www.jofem.org/index.php/jofem/article/viewArticle/1 5/15

'A systematic review of the potential herbal sources of future drugs effective in oxidant-related diseases.' https://www.ncbi.nlm.nih.gov/pubmed/19275687 (as accessed 2 Feb 2018).

'Effects of Nigella sativa and Thymoquinone on biochemical and subcellular changes in pancreatic β-cells of streptozotocin-induced diabetic rats' available from; https://www.ncbi.nlm.nih.gov/pubmed/20923501 (as accessed 29 Jan 2018).

'Insulinotropic properties of Nigella sativa oil in Streptozotocin plus Nicotinamide diabetic hamster' https://www.ncbi.nlm.nih.gov/pubmed/12443686 (as accessed 2 Feb 2018).

'Improvement of antihyperglycemic activity of Nano-Thymoquinone in rat model of type-2 diabetes' https://www.ncbi.nlm.nih.gov/pubmed/29421519 (as accessed 26 June 2018).

'Biochemical effects of Nigella sativa L seeds in diabetic rats.' https://www.ncbi.nlm.nih.gov/pubmed/16999030 (as accessed 2 Feb 2018).

'Effects of Nigella sativa on oxidative stress and beta-cell damage in streptozotocin-induced diabetic rats' https://www.ncbi.nlm.nih.gov/pubmed/15224410 (as accessed 2 Feb 2018).

'Nigella sativa seed extracts enhance glucose-induced insulin release from rat-isolated Langerhans islets' https://www.ncbi.nlm.nih.gov/pubmed/15482373 (as accessed 2 Feb 2018).

Hypoglycemic and Hypolipidemic Potential of Nigella sativa L. Seed Extract in Streptozotocin (STZ)-Induced Diabetic Rats' https://www.omicsonline.org/open-access/hypoglycemic-and-hypolipidemic-potential-of-nigella-sativa-l-seedextract-in-streptozotocin-stzinduced-diabetic-rats-2329-9029-1000158.php?aid=65796 (as accessed 2 Feb 2018).

'Antidiabetic Properties of a Spice Plant Nigella sativa' http://www.jofem.org/index.php/jofem/article/viewArticle/1 5/15 (as accessed 29 Jan 2018).

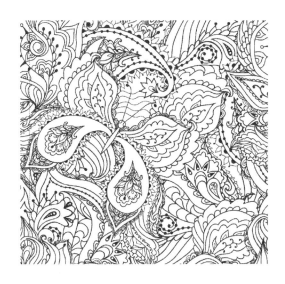

Chapter 10 - Drug Withdrawal and Brain Rewiring

Withdrawal from any substance is a hard slog. Not only are you dealing with the mental stress of changing habits, you are also having major negative physical symptoms too. If you are experiencing withdrawal from substances, I'm really sorry and I hope you get to feeling better ASAP. Yes, black cumin seed oil can help you!

What is Drug Withdrawal and Brain Rewiring?
Take hard, street drugs for even a short length of time and you are going to develop a problem that you will need to go through a withdrawal process from. Many pharmaceutical drugs will also require a withdrawal period, with doctors recommending the step-down approach to stopping drugs.

Street drug users are usually expected to withdraw from their addictions 'cold turkey' style. If either of those scenarios describe you or someone you love, then keep reading to find out how black seed oil can aid the process.

The Research

Remember to take it easy on yourself and be kind to you during this process. Yes, it's a process just like any other; it has a beginning, a middle and an end (with bragging rights after that!). So, a big good luck from me to you! :)

If you are having dreadful withdrawal symptoms, you might want to get your hands on some black cumin oil quickly. There are many different compounds in this oil that help many systems in the body. Black seed oil will also lessen your symptoms of withdrawal.

"Based on these results, it can be concluded that Thymoquinone prevents the development of tolerance and dependence to morphine." REF - 'Attenuation of morphine tolerance and dependence by Thymoquinone in mice'

"Nigella sativa extract affects conditioned place preference induced by morphine in rats" Meaning, the black seed extract lessened the pain of withdrawal.

"...also revealed that most of the therapeutic properties of this plant are due to the presence of Thymoquinone which is a major bioactive component of the essential oil." REF - 'Effect of Nigella sativa fixed oil on ethanol toxicity in rats'

Black Seed Oil for Alcohol Poisoning
A study published in 2014 showed that black seed oil reduced oxidative stress from alcohol poisoning in mice.

"This study showed that NSO may have protective effects against hepatotoxicity and renal toxicity of ethanol by decreasing lipid peroxidation and inflammation and preventing apoptosis." REF - 'Effect of Nigella sativa fixed oil on ethanol toxicity in rats'

"The results of the present study showed that the hydro-alcoholic extract of NS reduced the LPS-induced sickness behaviours in rats." REF - 'The effects of Nigella sativa on sickness behaviour induced by lipopolysaccharide in male Wistar rats'

Black Cumin for Opioid Dependence.
"Non-opioid drug, Nigella sativa, is effective in long-term treatment of opioid dependence. It not merely cures the opioid dependence but also cures the infections and weakness from which majority of addicts suffer." REF – 'A new and novel treatment of opioid dependence: Nigella sativa 500mg'

"As a conclusion, we would like to suggest probably with the supplementation of N. sativa to methadone, it will indirectly be a starting point to answer the question of opioid dependency and withdrawal..." REF - 'Opioid dependence and substitution therapy: Thymoquinone as potential novel supplement therapy for better outcome for methadone maintenance therapy substitution therapy'

Rewiring the Brain
The brain can be damaged by drugs, but another common way that the brain can be injured is through some sort of blunt force trauma called 'acquired brain injury'. Depending on how bad the acquired brain injury is, sometimes there is hope to rebuild those brains too.

There is much research suggesting that black cumin can play a part in regenerating brain cells. Previously, it has been thought that once certain parts of the brain were damaged, they couldn't become functional again.

Article 13, Volume 6, Issue 1, January 2016 of the Journal of Phytomedicine carried a research review which found that long-term administration of N. sativa increases 5-HT levels in the brain and improves learning and memory in rats. That's yet another study that gives hope to brain-injured people. They also had this to say, "Our literature review showed that NS and its components can be considered as promising agents in the treatment of nervous system disorders."
REF - Neuropharmacological effects of Nigella sativa'

"Based on these results, it can be concluded that Thymoquinone prevents the development of tolerance and dependence to morphine." REF - 'Attenuation of morphine tolerance and dependence by Thymoquinone in mice'

If your brain is in recovery after a drug addiction or brain injury of any kind, black seed oil is a great way to get back some of those precious cells.

References
'Attenuation of morphine tolerance and dependence by Thymoquinone in mice'
https://www.researchgate.net/publication/303748914 (as accessed Jan 29, 2018).

'Effect of Nigella sativa fixed oil on ethanol toxicity in rats'
https://www.researchgate.net/publication/274722955 (as accessed 9 Feb 2018).

'The effects of Nigella sativa on sickness behaviour induced by lipopolysaccharide in male Wistar rats'
https://pdfs.semanticscholar.org/f1ac/846b7de2d627efb5a7c9 86153cf42ee3ae7e.pdf (as accessed 9 Feb 2018).

'Opioid dependence and substitution therapy: Thymoquinone as potential novel supplement therapy for better outcome for methadone maintenance therapy substitution therapy'
https://europepmc.org/articles/PMC4387227 (as accessed 9 Feb 2018).

'A new and novel treatment of opioid dependence: Nigella

sativa 500mg'
http://www.ayubmed.edu.pk/JAMC/PAST/20-2/Sangi.pdf
(as accessed 9 Feb 2018).

'Attenuation of morphine tolerance and dependence by
Thymoquinone in mice'
https://www.ncbi.nlm.nih.gov/pmc/articles/PMC4884218 (as
accessed 9 Feb 2018).

'A review on therapeutic potential of Nigella sativa: A
miracle herb'
https://www.ncbi.nlm.nih.gov/pmc/articles/PMC3642442/ (as
accessed 9 Feb 2018).

'Neuropharmacological effects of Nigella sativa'
http://ajp.mums.ac.ir/article_6231.html (as accessed 9 Feb
2018).
Perveen T, Abdullah A, Haider S, Sonia B, Munawar AS,
Haleem DJ. Long-term administration of Nigella sativa
affects nociception and improves learning and memory in
rats. Pak J Biochem Mol Biol. 2008;41(3):141–143

'Running Triggers VGF-Mediated Oligodendrogenesis to
Prolong the Lifespan of Snf2h-Null Ataxic Mice.' Published
11 October 2016 issue of Journal "Cell Reports" by Prof
David J. Picketts, Dr Matías Alvarez-Saavedra and others.

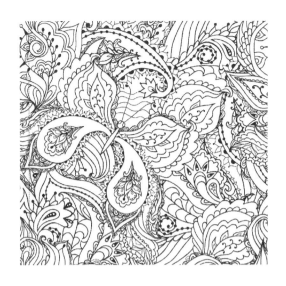

Chapter 11 – Enemas

The official name for what we are talking about here is Anuvasana Basti, which simply means enemas with medicated oils, tonics and/or herbal milks.

What are Enemas?
In our modern world of fast 'food' and imbalanced diets, is it any wonder that the use of enemas is on the rise? Basically, an enema is the insertion of liquid into the lower bowel via the rectum, in an effort to dislodge the faeces that doesn't want to exit on its own accord. Hold the liquid for as long as you can (up to half an hour), then expel. Don't worry if you can't hold for that long because even just a few minutes on the first time will get things going. Then follow up with another with the aim of holding it for longer.

The Research

Enemas are one of the classical detoxification (Panchakarma) therapies and indicated for use in all Ayurvedic Vata disorders.

Enemas are best performed when a person is not suffering from things like breathing trouble or coughing and you must not have any complications of a gastrointestinal type. Enemas are NOT recommended after the 7th month of pregnancy either.

When Asthapana Basti is given to those who are physically weak or debilitated, or in the presence of hunger, thirst or fatigue, the vasti remedies will produce further irritation and may even be deadly.

I recommend always having a support person nearby while having an enema, especially for the first few times. The effect is usually sudden and can cause you to become faint.

People NOT Suited to Having Enemas

Each person's physical situation is different and those that are unsuited to having an enema would be:

- Pandu – anaemia,
- Kamala – jaundice
- Meha – diabetes, urinary tract disorders
- Peenasa – rhinitis
- Niranna – on an empty stomach

- Pleeha - disease of the spleen, Splenomegaly
- Vid bhedi – diarrhoea
- Guru koshta – hard bowels - constipated
- Kaphodara – Kapha type of Ascites
- Abhishyandi a type of eye disorder
- Bhrusha Sthula – profound obesity
- Krumi Koshta – intestinal worm infestation
- Adhyamaruta – gout

In addition, those that are suffering from artificial poison, goiter, filariasis or scrofula should also avoid having an enema. REF - 'Niruha basti Panchakarma method, benefits, side effects, management'

Black Seed Oil Enema Recipe
In a pot, warm together the following:
- 5-10 drops black cumin seed oil
- 4 oz. organic raw honey
- 4 oz. warm sesame oil
- 4 oz. warm purified water
(4 oz. = about 120ml)

Mix together very well, administer the enema, and retain for at least 15 minutes or longer if possible. The mixture should be warm when using.

References
'Niruha basti Panchakarma method, benefits, side effects, management' https://easyayurveda.com/2016/08/20/niruha-

basti-panchakarma-method-benefits-side-effects/ (as accessed 12 Feb 2018).

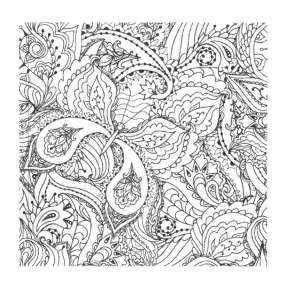

Chapter 12 - Epilepsy

There have been promising results from the most recent findings when it comes to treating epilepsy with black seed oil.

What is Epilepsy?
Up until about the last couple of hundred years, a person suffering from epilepsy was thought to be possessed by demons. We now know it stems from neurological problems characterized by seizures. Epileptic seizures are episodes that can vary all the way from brief and nearly undetectable periods to long periods of full body, vigorous shaking.

The Research
From an Iranian university's medical sciences department research, I found this comment on a study of black seed oil

vs epilepsy, "The mean frequency of seizures decreased significantly during treatment with extract (p<0.05). It can be concluded that the water extract of Nigella sativa has anti-epileptic effects in children with refractory seizures" REF -' The effect of Nigella sativa L. (black cumin seed) on intractable pediatric seizures'

"NS oil was demonstrated to be effective in preventing pentylenetetrazole (PTZ)-induced seizures compared to valproate." And, "These results indicate that Thymoquinone may have anticonvulsant activity in the petit mal epilepsy probably through an opioid receptor-mediated increase in GABAergic tone."

And, "Experimental studies have demonstrated potential anticonvulsant and potent antioxidant effects of NS oil in reducing oxidative stress, excitability, and the induction of seizures in epileptic animals besides ameliorating certain adverse effects of antiepileptic drugs." REF - 'Anticonvulsant effects of Thymoquinone, the major constituent of Nigella sativa seeds, in mice.'

"So, it could be concluded that the treatment with CFX induced imbalance between the excitatory and the inhibitory amino acids which may lead to the initiation of epileptic seizures and the treatment with NS was found to ameliorate these neurological defects which reflect its potent antiepileptic activity." - REF - 'Potential role of Nigella sativa (black cumin) in epilepsy.'

References

Akhondian, Javad & Parsa, Ali & Rakhshande, Hassan. (2008). 'The effect of Nigella sativa L. (black cumin seed) on intractable pediatric seizures' Medical science monitor: international medical journal of experimental and clinical research. 13. CR555-9.
https://www.researchgate.net/publication/5799395

Hosseinzadeh H, Parvardeh S. 'Anticonvulsant effects of Thymoquinone, the major constituent of Nigella sativa seeds, in mice' Phytomedicine 2004;11:56-64.
https://www.sciencedirect.com/science/article/pii/S0944711304702950

'Potential role of Nigella sativa (black cumin) in epilepsy.' Int J Nutr Pharmacol Neurol Dis [serial online] 2014 [cited 2018 Jan 24]; 4:188-9.
http://www.ijnpnd.com/text.asp?2014/4/3/188/132680

'Evaluation of the possible epileptogenic activity of ciprofloxacin: the role of Nigella sativa on amino acids neurotransmitters.' Arafa et al. Jazan University.

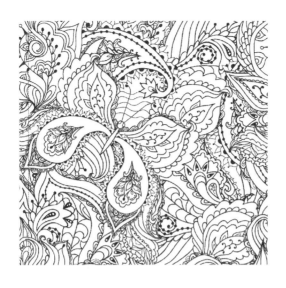

Chapter 13 – Estrogen

There is plenty of research to suggest that black cumin oil has estrogen-like effects, and is helpful in regulating hormones, especially in those women experiencing menopause.

What is Estrogen?
Estrogen is important for both men and women but is more prevalent in women's health. Estrogens are the name given to a group of sex hormones, namely; estrone, estradiol, and estriol. Estrogens play essential roles in the regulation of the menstrual cycle and reproductive system and they also regulate the growth and development of female secondary sexual characteristics, such as breasts, pubic and armpit hair. Dear Reader, if you are a woman coping as best as you can with dropping estrogen levels during menopause, black seed

oil may offer you a little relief from these symptoms. Because this is a subject close to my own heart at this time, I've also included a chapter dedicated specifically to menopause.

Men also have estrogen in their bodies but not as much as women. Teens and young men have high levels of testosterone and low levels of estrogen. As men age, testosterone gets converted into estrogens due to the aromatase reaction. Aromatase is mostly found in fat cells, so the more body fat a man has, especially around the midsection, the more aromatase and hence the more estrogen will be converted.

The Research

"These data suggest that N. sativa possesses an estrogenic function in the ovariectomized rat model which can be helpful in managing menopausal symptoms as an alternative for Hormone Replacement Therapy"

and...

"The results demonstrated that N. sativa exert estrogenic effect were exhibited through uterotrophic assay and vaginal cell cornification as well as blood estrogen level. Furthermore, low dose N. sativa, methanol extract and linoleic acid had prominent estrogenic-like effects which were significantly different from those of the control group in different experiments." REF – 'Assessing estrogenic activity of Nigella sativa in ovariectomized rats using vaginal cornification assay'

"The findings indicated the probable beneficial role for N. sativa in the treatment of postmenopausal symptoms and possibility of using N. sativa as an alternative to hormone replacement therapy (HRT) for post menopause in humans." REF - 'Effect of Nigella sativa on reproductive system in experimental menopause rat model'

Here is another heads up on black seed oil's potential to aid those with dropping estrogen levels; "The methanol extracts of Derris reticulata and Dracaena lourieri showed the most potent estrogenic activity on both estrogen-receptor subtypes, while, the methanol extracts of Butea monosperma, Erythrina fusca, and Dalbergia candenatensis revealed significant estrogenic activity on ERβ only. Nigella sativa, Sophora japonica, Artabotrys harmandii, and Clitorea hanceana showed estrogenic effect only after naringinase treatment. The most potent antiestrogenic effect was revealed by Aframomum melegueta, Dalbergia candenatensis, Dracena loureiri, and Mansonia gagei." REF - 'Screening for estrogenic and antiestrogenic activities of plants growing in Egypt and Thailand'

There is so much research on this subject that it seems ridiculous to turn to synthetic drugs to assist dropping estrogen levels.

"Thymoquinone, a phytochemical compound found in plant Nigella sativa, has been shown anti-cancer effects via regulation of apoptosis, estrogen metabolism, MAPK and Akt signalling pathways in breast cancer." - REF - 'Role of dietary bioactive natural products in estrogen receptor-positive breast cancer'

"The main cause of osteoporosis is menopause or estrogen-deficiency. Nigella sativa reverses osteoporosis in ovariectomized rats, which could be attributed to its high content of unsaturated fatty acids as well as its antioxidant and anti-inflammatory properties." - REF - 'Nigella Sativa reverses osteoporosis in ovariectomized rats'

"...low dose N. sativa, methanol extract and linoleic acid had prominent estrogenic-like effects which were significantly different from those of control group (p<0.05) in different experiments." - REF - 'Effect of Nigella sativa on reproductive system in experimental menopause rat model'

"Treatment with N. sativa induced a significant reduction of prevalence and severity of menopausal symptoms as well as significant improvement in some components of quality of life." - REF - 'Alternative supplement for enhancement of reproductive health and metabolic profile among perimenopausal women: a novel role of Nigella sativa'

As you can see, black cumin seed oil does give some hope of riding out the menopause hurricane with a bit more grace (I know it has for me!).

References

'Assessing estrogenic activity of Nigella sativa in ovariectomized rats using vaginal cornification assay' https://www.researchgate.net/publication/228624865 (as accessed 26 Feb 2018).

'Effect of Nigella sativa on reproductive system in experimental menopause rat model' https://www.researchgate.net/publication/287269213 (as accessed 26 Feb 2018).

'Screening for estrogenic and antiestrogenic activities of plants growing in Egypt and Thailand' https://www.ncbi.nlm.nih.gov/pmc/articles/PMC3129019/ (as accessed 26 Feb 2018).

'Role of dietary bioactive natural products in estrogen receptor-positive breast cancer' https://www.ncbi.nlm.nih.gov/pmc/articles/PMC5033666/ (as accessed 26 Feb 2018).

'Nigella Sativa reverses osteoporosis in ovariectomized rats' https://www.ncbi.nlm.nih.gov/pmc/articles/PMC3898005/ (as accessed 26 Feb 2018).

'Effect of Nigella sativa on reproductive system in experimental menopause rat model' https://www.ncbi.nlm.nih.gov/pmc/articles/PMC4884222/ (as

accessed 26 Feb 2018).

'Alternative supplement for enhancement of reproductive health and metabolic profile among perimenopausal women: a novel role of Nigella sativa' https://www.ncbi.nlm.nih.gov/pmc/articles/PMC4387233/ (as accessed 26 Feb 2018).

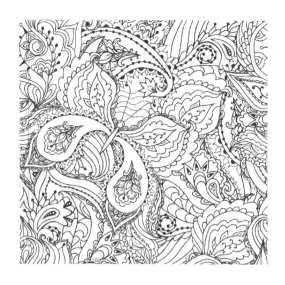

Chapter 14 – Fibromyalgia

I found exactly zero research studies connecting fibromyalgia (FM) with black cumin. However, I did find some useful information about it in my research travels.

What is Fibromyalgia?

If you are a fibro sufferer, then I don't need to insert the full rundown of all the points of pain and everything else that goes along with it. However, did you know one of the more bizarre aspects of fibromyalgia is that it appears to manifest in conjunction with or after the onset of a few different viral infections, one of which is known as Epstein Barr Virus?

According to the CDC, it is a type of herpes virus that they say most people contract at some point throughout their lives, though fibromyalgia sufferers tend to experience more painful and frequent symptoms than those with the virus alone.

There are around 17 common viruses that often circulate throughout human populations, but Epstein Barr is almost always present in fibromyalgia patients (also with a handful of other viruses such as rotavirus and other strains of herpes).

Surely then, one way to avoid getting fibromyalgia is to avoid getting these viruses? I'm sure you can see the value in taking a natural antiviral substance such as black seed oil to assist with not only avoiding fibromyalgia in the first place but also for the analgesic effect to relieve pain symptoms in the event that you do have fibro.

The Research
Often treated with Tramadol painkillers, fibromyalgia sufferers should be aware of the potential liver damage that can occur with long-term use of this drug. You need to ease the pain but not at the expense of your liver or kidneys!

The study titled, 'Effect of Nigella sativa Linn oil on tramadol-induced hepato - and nephrotoxicity in adult male albino rats' tells us, "Many medicinal properties have been attributed to NsL oil seed extract and/or its oil, including antihistaminic, antihypertensive, analgesic, anti-inflammatory, hypoglycemic, antibacterial, antifungal, antitumour as well as protective effects against hepatotoxicity and nephrotoxicity." REF - 'Effect of Nigella sativa Linn oil on tramadol-induced hepato - and nephrotoxicity in adult male albino rats'

Because I was unable to source a lot of information relating fibromyalgia to black cumin, I decided to include what information I could find, regardless of the fact that it has nothing to do with the subject of this book.

Exercise

I know, I know, you have heard this before, but really, exercise beats a LOT of different pharmaceuticals, hands down. It should be moderate exercise and doesn't need to be aerobic or strenuous in nature. A research review found that "A systematic review of various exercise trials including a total of 2494 patients indicates that exercise overall shows significant effects in reducing pain and related FM symptoms. At least moderate level of exercise intensity is considered necessary to produce appreciative benefit. However, recent evidence suggests that various mind/body exercises that do not require strenuous movement or raising the heart rate may help reduce FM symptoms. For example, group qigong exercise, tai chi exercise and yoga practice showed significantly greater symptomatic improvement compared with the patients in the control group or waitlist. A meta-analysis reports medium to high effect size in pain reduction from these exercises for FM."

In the same paper, we find, "Another RCT evaluating mindfulness exercise has shown significant improvement in social and emotional functioning. Thus, this type of therapeutic effort may not necessarily improve pain but still may positively impact some important life domains of FM patients."
REF – 'Management of fibromyalgia syndrome in 2016'

Hyperbaric Oxygen Therapy
More studies need to be done but hyperbaric oxygen therapy (HBOT) has given some good results so far for the relief of pain symptoms in FM patients. "The HBOT was five 90 sessions per week for 8 weeks, which showed significant symptom reduction and some normalization of neural activity based upon SPECT imaging. However, it is noteworthy that patients often complained of symptom worsening during the first 4 weeks. This study also could not blind patients. Although the results are promising, HBOT is not a benign approach; it carries a risk of oxygen toxicity and other side effects." REF - 'Management of fibromyalgia syndrome in 2016'

Transcranial Stimulation
This is a grasping-at-straws idea, but, "TMS may modulate mood but the effects on pain may be marginal." REF - 'Review Repetitive Transcranial Magnetic Stimulation for Fibromyalgia: Systematic Review and Meta-Analysis'

If you are at your wits end with the pain, then there are a

few more experimental therapies described in the reference links.

References

'Management of fibromyalgia syndrome in 2016'
https://www.ncbi.nlm.nih.gov/pmc/articles/PMC5066139/ (as accessed 1 Feb 2018).

'Efficacy of different types of aerobic exercise in fibromyalgia syndrome: a systematic review and meta-analysis of randomised controlled trials'
https://www.ncbi.nlm.nih.gov/pubmed/20459730/ (as accessed 1 Feb 2018).

'Exercise Therapy for Fibromyalgia'
https://www.ncbi.nlm.nih.gov/pmc/articles/PMC3165132/ as accessed 1 Feb 2018).

'A comprehensive review of 46 exercise treatment studies in fibromyalgia (1988-2005)'
https://www.ncbi.nlm.nih.gov/pubmed/16999856/ (as accessed 1 Feb 2018).

'Efficacy and effectiveness of exercise on tender points in adults with fibromyalgia: a meta-analysis of randomized controlled trials.'
https://www.ncbi.nlm.nih.gov/pubmed/22046512/ (as accessed 1 Feb 2018).

'A randomized controlled trial of 8-form Tai chi improves

symptoms and functional mobility in fibromyalgia patients'
https://www.ncbi.nlm.nih.gov/pubmed/22581278/ (as
accessed 1 Feb 2018).

'A randomized trial of tai chi for fibromyalgia'
https://www.ncbi.nlm.nih.gov/pubmed/20818876/ (as
accessed 1 Feb 2018).

'A pilot randomized controlled trial of the Yoga of
Awareness program in the management of fibromyalgia'
https://www.ncbi.nlm.nih.gov/pubmed/20946990/ (as
accessed 1 Feb 2018).

'Effect of Nigella sativa Linn oil on tramadol-induced
hepato- and nephrotoxicity in adult male albino rats'
https://www.ncbi.nlm.nih.gov/pmc/articles/PMC5598165/ (as
accessed 31 Jan 2018).

'Complementary and alternative exercise for fibromyalgia: a
meta-analysis'
https://www.ncbi.nlm.nih.gov/pubmed/23569397/ (as
accessed 1 Feb 2018).

'Review Repetitive Transcranial Magnetic Stimulation for
Fibromyalgia: Systematic Review and Meta-Analysis'
https://www.ncbi.nlm.nih.gov/pubmed/25581213/ (as
accessed 1 Feb 2018).

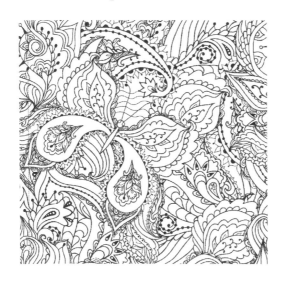

Chapter 15 – Grey Hair

Mix together an equal amount of olive oil and black cumin seed oil and massage it into the scalp. Wash out with warm water after an hour. Repeat about once a month for soft, shiny and healthy hair. This routine also promotes the growth of new hair follicles!

What is Grey Hair?

You know when your kids stress you out for decades on end, then you look in the mirror and say, "What colour is my hair?" Well, THAT'S grey hair. But seriously, the hair goes grey because it loses pigment, usually, as we age. They haven't yet figured out why that happens.

Contained in the skin coatings of black cumin seeds is approximately 15% melanin, one of the main ingredients that gives the hair colour.

"The key enzyme of the melanin synthesis pathway is tyrosinase."

"...natural plant melanins extracted from e.g. Nigella sativa, have interesting effects on mammalian cells"

The Research
"Depigmenting agents and those increasing melanin synthesis are used in medicine and cosmetology. Also, natural plant melanins extracted from Nigella sativa, for example, have interesting effects on mammalian cells." REF - 'Factors affecting melanogenesis and methods used for identification of pigmentation disorders'

"Recently, melanin was known to exist in the outer coat of the N. sativa seeds which represents around 15% of the seed coat alone" - 'Cytotoxicity assay for herbal melanin derived from Nigella sativa seeds using in vitro cell lines'

References
'Cytotoxicity assay for herbal melanin derived from Nigella sativa seeds using in vitro cell lines'
http://www.iosrjournals.org/iosr-jhss/papers/Vol.%2022%20Issue10/Version-5/G2210054351.pdf (as accessed 2 June 2018).

'Factors affecting melanogenesis and methods used for

identification of pigmentation disorders'
https://www.ncbi.nlm.nih.gov/pubmed/18942345 (as
accessed 2 June 2018).

Grey Hair

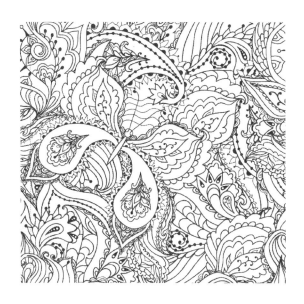

Chapter 16 – Gut Health

"If ya' don't eat, ya' don't shit. If ya' don't shit, ya' die"
Yes, gut health is that important!

What is Gut Health?
A healthy gut is a moving gut. Once things slow down in that department, the gut troubles will start. From mild to life-threatening, the problems that can arise are wildly varied in severity. Maintain a healthy gut and gastrointestinal system and you'll be maintaining a healthy body from the gut out.

The Research
One of the most common causes of stomach and duodenal ulcers is the Helicobacter pylori infection. A research study

involving more plant species than just the black seed found that it does indeed aid in getting rid of this infection. "...most potent urease inhibitory was observed for Zingiber officinale, Laurus nobilis, and Nigella sativa with IC50 values of 48.54, 48.69 and 59.10 µg/mL, respectively" (IC50 refers to the half maximal inhibitory concentration is a measure of the potency of a substance in inhibiting a specific biological or biochemical function.) REF - 'Screening of 20 commonly used Iranian traditional medicinal plants against urease'

On the way to replacing pharma drugs, perhaps? ... "TQ, especially the high dose level, corrected the altered parameters in a comparable manner to that of the reference drug used, omeprazole." REF - 'Thymoquinone: Novel gastroprotective mechanisms'

The worst thing that can occur in the gut is cancer. There's a black seed oil research paper for that... "These results, which provide molecular evidence both in vitro and in vivo, support our conclusion that Thymoquinone can activate caspase-3 and caspase-9 and thus result in the chemosensitisation of gastric cancer cells to 5-FU-induced cell death." REF - 'Thymoquinone inhibits growth and augments 5-fluorouracil-induced apoptosis in gastric cancer cells both in vitro and in vivo'

References

'Screening of 20 commonly used Iranian traditional medicinal plants against urease' https://www.ncbi.nlm.nih.gov/pubmed/24711846 (as accessed 26 June 2018).

'Thymoquinone: Novel gastroprotective mechanisms' https://www.ncbi.nlm.nih.gov/pubmed/23051678 (as accessed 26 June 2018).

'Thymoquinone inhibits growth and augments 5-fluorouracil-induced apoptosis in gastric cancer cells both in vitro and in vivo' https://www.ncbi.nlm.nih.gov/pubmed/22206670 (as accessed 26 June 2018).

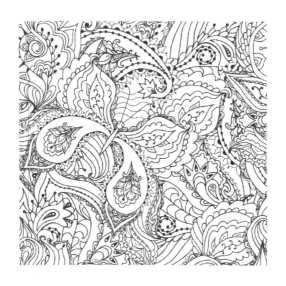

Chapter 17 – Hair Growth

Hair loss can occur for many reasons like microbial infection, inflammatory conditions, aging and chemotherapy just to name a few. Thankfully, it's black seed oil to the rescue once again.

The few studies that have been done in this area have produced outstanding results when testing the effects of the mighty black cumin seed for hair regrowth. The first study was on twenty patients affected by Telogen Effluvium (TE) in a double-blind, placebo-controlled and randomized study.

What is Hair Growth?
Hair on the human body grows in 3 stages; Anagen phase (growth), Catagen phase (transitional, renewal) and Telogen

phase (resting, shedding). One of the more important chemical compounds in hair growth is melanin for the colour, as discussed in the previous chapter on grey hair.

In addition, "The homeostasis of the epidermis and hair follicle is primarily regulated by the cellular interaction between keratinocytes and melanocytes"

In 2013, sufferers of Telogen Effluvium received some hope in the form of a published paper, 'Evaluation of a Therapeutic Alternative for Telogen Effluvium: A Pilot Study' in which 70% of the 20 participants in a placebo study achieved significant hair growth results using a mere 0.5% strength of Nigella sativa oil, daily for 3 months. That is a very low strength oil, so with a stronger oil, which is pretty much all on the market, hair growth should improve even more. What a wonderful side effect if you are taking this wonder oil for any other ailment. And, if you are taking it directly for hair growth, what a wonderful gift this oil is even beyond the direct healing of your hair.

The Research
The results were nothing less than amazing! 70% of the participants in the control group showed significant improvement in hair regrowth. That's not too shabby in my book! REF - 'Prostaglandin D2 inhibits hair growth and is elevated in bald scalp of men with androgenetic alopecia'

"Videodermatoscopic analysis showed a significant

increment of hair density and hair thickness in patients treated with NS. NS was also able to reduce the inflammation observed in the majority of patients affected by TE" REF - 'Prostaglandin D2 inhibits hair growth and is elevated in bald scalp of men with androgenetic alopecia'

My own black cumin seed oil story includes the bonus of thicker hair. By the time I first started taking the oil, I'd lost about 50-60% of my hair through menopause. Since taking this oil, I've regained about 20% of what I'd lost.

Researchers in Bangladesh tested coconut oil against an oil mix with Nigella sativa for hair regrowth and in the researcher's own words, "...the present study can give a tremendous solution in the field of hair fall it can be said that hair fall is stopped." REF – 'Formulation and finding out the efficacy of the herbal hair oil over simple coconut oil (purified)'

In a rat study on chemotherapy-induced alopecia, it was found, "...it is evident that N. sativa provides significant protection against chemotherapy-induced alopecia." Now that's pretty exciting seeing as chemotherapy-induced alopecia can be quite severe and usually taking many months or years to regrow without help. REF - 'Protective role of Nigella sativa in chemotherapy-induced alopecia'

Anecdotal Evidence

"I strongly advise you to use black seed oil (A.K.A Black cumin seed, Kalonji, Nigella Sativa), I swear to god this is the strongest topical I ever tried. It stopped my hair loss in a few days as it inhibits the crth2 pathway for pgd2, lowers TNF alpha, 5ar inhibitor and lowers androgen receptors."

"I lost all body hair too, including eyebrows and eyelashes. I also stopped sweating for two whole years! I only realized that as soon as I started taking black seeds, the day after I was sweating whilst hoovering. My immune system was out of order. But I started taking 7 black seeds with Manuka honey mixed in warm water. Alhumdulillah my eyebrows are back and my eyelashes. My body hair too."

"Anyway, as for my bald scalp, it's still curing. I used a combination of black seed oil and olive oil too on my head, not too much as I had severe eczema on my scalp.
Now I have about 60-70% of my head hair. Some are at the initial stages and have just popped out. The doctors had given little hope and said there's no medication for alopecia!!!"

References

'Prostaglandin D2 inhibits hair growth and is elevated in bald scalp of men with androgenetic alopecia'
https://www.researchgate.net/publication/276493673

'Formulation and finding out the efficacy of the herbal hair oil over simple coconut oil (purified)' Dulal et al., IJPSR, 2014; Vol. 5(5): 1801-1805.

http://immortalhair.forumandco.com/t9304-estrogen-dominance

'Protective role of Nigella sativa in chemotherapy-induced alopecia'
Uzma Saleem et al. Bangladesh Journal of Pharmacology 2017; 12: 455-462.

Hair Growth

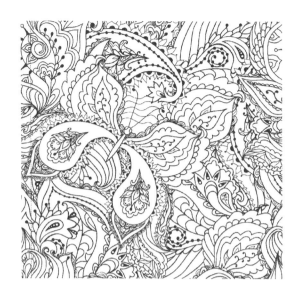

Chapter 18 - Hepatitis C (HCV)

With Hepatitis C becoming wildly prevalent, the WHO statistics speak for themselves. It was estimated in 2017 that globally, "71 million people have a chronic hepatitis C infection" and "...die mostly from cirrhosis and hepatocellular carcinoma." REF – WHO Hepatitis C

What is Hepatitis C?
A blood-borne liver disease describes Hepatitis C. The severity of which varies dramatically from nearly nothing to serious and life-long with eventual fatal complications. This disease is normally spread via blood contamination of shared syringes or unprotected sex.

The Research

In 2013 in Egypt, there was a study done on 30 patients where the researchers evaluated the safety, efficacy and tolerability of Nigella sativa (N. sativa) in patients with Hepatitis C that were not eligible for interferon. Many people were excluded for several reasons, including having any other type of Hepatitis or hepatocellular carcinoma or other cancers. They also excluded those with a major severe illness and those that had a history of treatment non-compliance.

Over the course of 3 months, the participants were dosed at 450 mg three times daily. The conclusion of that study was, "N. sativa administration in patients with hepatitis C virus (HCV) was tolerable, safe, decreased viral load, and improved oxidative stress" REF - 'Effects of Nigella sativa on outcome of hepatitis C in Egypt'

Oxidative stress is one of the main causes of liver injury. It depletes the antioxidant enzymes sources and lowers the ability of cells to function against injury. Major liver damage can be induced by oxidative stress caused by the Hepatitis virus.

An Indian product made from black seed oil called Alpha-Zam was tested against Hepatitis C and the researcher's conclusion was, "Alpha-zam selectively inhibits HCV replication and therefore has the potential for a novel antiviral agent against HCV infection." REF - 'Selective

Inhibition of Hepatitis C Virus Replication by Alpha-Zam, a Nigella sativa Seed Formulation'

While it's not quite Hepatitis C, liver injury is the common denominator, so I thought this next paper would be of interest too. In 2008, they knew that black seed oil helps to protect and repair the liver. "Our results suggest that Nigella sativa treatment protects the rat liver against to hepatic ischemia-reperfusion injury." REF - 'Nigella sativa relieves the deleterious effects of ischemia-reperfusion injury on liver'

References
WHO – Hepatitis C - http://www.who.int/en/news-room/fact-sheets/detail/hepatitis-c (as accessed 21 June 2018).

'Effects of Nigella sativa on outcome of hepatitis C in Egypt' https://www.ncbi.nlm.nih.gov/pmc/articles/PMC3646144/ (as accessed 21 June 2018).

'Selective Inhibition of Hepatitis C Virus Replication by Alpha-Zam, a Nigella sativa Seed Formulation' https://www.ncbi.nlm.nih.gov/pmc/articles/PMC5412185/ (as accessed 21 June 2018).

'Nigella sativa relieves the deleterious effects of ischemia-reperfusion injury on liver' - https://www.ncbi.nlm.nih.gov/pubmed/18777598/ (as accessed 21 June 2018).

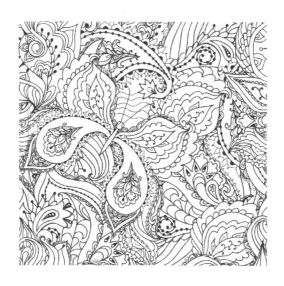

Chapter 19 – High Blood Pressure

You can go the pharma route and take diuretics, ACE inhibitors, angiotensin II receptor blockers (ARBs), calcium channel blockers, beta blockers or renin inhibitors, all of which will make you sicker in the long run. Do you know the side effects of the drugs you are taking? I hope so.

What is High Blood Pressure?
High blood pressure (hypertension) is usually a long-term medical condition in which the blood pressure in the arteries is persistently elevated. This condition does not usually cause symptoms but it's not good for your body to have elevated blood pressure for extended periods of time. It can cause complications like increasing the risk of heart disease, stroke, and even death.

Researchers now think that there is evidence suggesting that hypertension may be attributable to the increased production of reactive oxygen species (ROS).

"Oxidative stress occurs when there is an imbalance between the generation of reactive oxygen species (ROS) and the antioxidant defence systems so that the latter become overwhelmed" REF - Implications of oxidative stress and homocysteinein the pathophysiology of essential hypertension'

The Research

You may have to stay on the pharma drugs while you test out black cumin seed oil to see if you are one of the lucky ones that can treat high blood pressure with this healing oil. Always consult your health professional for advice on how to do this. If they won't incorporate natural healing into their repertoire, then you need a new health professional.

Late in 2016, a review was undertaken looking at many published studies into black cumin seed in relation to high blood pressure and the researchers found, "Our meta-analysis suggests that short-term treatment with N. sativa powder can significantly reduce blood pressure levels" -

In a survey of some of the plants used in traditional treatment of hypertension and diabetes in South-East Morocco, N. sativa was the plant most frequently used by medical herbalists and others." REF - 'Pharmacological and toxicological properties of Nigella sativa.'

The researchers don't quite know yet why black cumin seed helps hypertension but they suspect it is the combination of the "...cardiac depressant, diuretic, calcium channel blockade, and antioxidant properties" In the same review article, it was found that "NS is a promising medicinal plant with many therapeutic properties." REF - 'Nigella sativa and Its Protective Role in Oxidative Stress and Hypertension'

I found more than 11 other animal research study papers that have shown significant effects gained from black seed oil against hypertension.

References

'Pharmacological and toxicological properties of Nigella sativa.'
https://www.ncbi.nlm.nih.gov/pubmed/28195061 (as accessed 26 Jan 2018)

'Nigella Sativa and Its Protective Role in Oxidative Stress and Hypertension' - Evidence-Based Complementary and Alternative Medicine 2013 (2013): 1–9.

'Implications of oxidative stress and homocysteinein the pathophysiology of essential hypertension' - Journal of Cardiovascular Pharmacology vol. 42, no. 4, pp. 453-461, 2003.

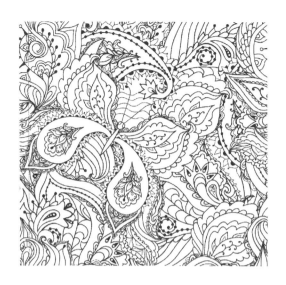

Chapter 20 - How to Grow and/or Cold Press Your Own Oil

If you are anything like me, then you will want to grow your own so you can carefully monitor the entire process of your oil from go to whoa. Sometimes it's a challenge to grow what you want, but black seed, the wondrous Nigella sativa, is endemic to the Middle East region of the world, meaning that if it's hot where you are, you can certainly have a successful crop of black seeds.

The most potent and medicinally important seeds originate from Egypt.

If you want to grow your own, you will yield the best results if you live in a hot dry region, mimicking the climate of

Egypt with an average yearly rainfall of 24.7ml (0.972in). Of course, that's after babying the baby seedlings into medium-sized plants.

Nigella sativa is an annual plant that grows from 15 to 60 cm tall. Nigella blooms in the summer with pink, white or blue flowers and has attractive feathered leaves.

Sowing

You can start to sow black seeds just before the last frost of spring.

For outside sowing space, 20-30cm (10-12 inches) apart and if you are sowing indoors, it's best to use peat pots to retain the moisture required to feed those thirsty seedlings when they arrive. Germination time is 2-3 weeks. Temperature 21°C (70°F).

Transplanting

Transplant outdoors following the last frost or in autumn or at about 7-8 weeks of age.

Nigella likes full sunlight and good to great drainage with a soil pH of 6-7.

Water Requirements

Once these plants are established, you just water during very dry spells.

What is Cold Pressing?

Whether you grow your own or just buy organic packets of black cumin seeds, the next step is cold pressing. ***What is the difference between cold pressing and other types of oil extraction methods?

Cold pressing is better than heat methods of oil extraction because ALL the goodness is retained and nothing is heated out of the final product = every single healing molecule is retained.

The Research

The cold-pressed oil process can be achieved at home with a motorized or hand-crank expeller press. It's one of those ye olde manual jobs that, if you let it, can bring you kind of 'closer' to the food you are consuming. The cold press comes with instructions on how to use it. You just put the seeds in the top, a glass jar at the bottom and crank the handle and wallah! ...100% fresh black seed oil is yours!

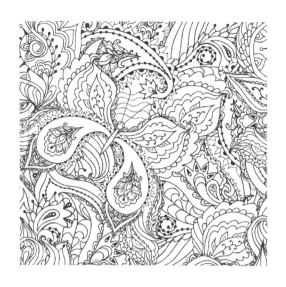

Chapter 21 - Immune System and Colds/Influenza

What are Colds/Influenza?

Colds and influenza (the flu) are two very different sicknesses. A cold is a bacterial infection that gives you a runny nose, sneezing and coughing, and a flu is apparently a viral infection and has the same general symptoms of a cold.

As I'm sure you already know, our body fights off invading bacteria and viruses with our vastly complex immune system. What you might not know is how an immunomodulator helps the immune system.

Merriam-Webster tells us that an immunomodulator is "...a substance that affects the functioning of the immune system" and there is a plethora of evidence that black seed oil does indeed affect the functioning of the human immune system. Runny noses and stuffy head colds would be in grave danger of being wiped out if everyone used black seed oil.

The Research

A study was conducted to investigate the effect of Nigella sativa on hormone reproduction and thyroid function in female rats. The result revealed a significant increase in levels of LH, Estrogen T3 and T4 and a significant decrease in levels of TSH. - 'A review on therapeutic potential of Nigella sativa: A miracle herb'

Research suggestive of enhanced immune response. REF - 'Nigella sativa: effect on human lymphocytes and polymorphonuclear leukocyte phagocytic activity' Immunopharmacology. 1995; 30 (2): 147-155 .

"Results demonstrated that the aqueous extract of N. sativa significantly enhances splenocyte proliferation in a dose-responsive manner. In addition, the aqueous extract of N. sativa favours the secretion of Th2, versus Th1, cytokines by splenocytes." What did that mean? Well, cytokines are regulatory proteins that are released by cells of the immune system and act as intercellular mediators in the generation of an immune response. They are immunomodulating agents and splenocytes are any white blood cells in the spleen. The black seed increased the production of white blood cells in the spleen AND the cellular communications! REF - 'A review on therapeutic potential of Nigella sativa: A miracle herb'

In another rat study from 2011, black seed oil was proven to aid the immune system yet again. In a 5-dose treatment protocol, the black seed enhanced both the total white blood cells count and bone marrow cellularity "...significantly" "These results confirmed the immunomodulatory activity of black seed, and may have therapeutical implications in prophylactic treatment of opportunistic infections and as supportive treatment in oncogenic cases" REF - 'Evaluation of immunomodulatory effect of three herbal plants growing in Egypt'

In 2012, researchers declared, "We demonstrate that N. sativa seed extract significantly improves symptoms and immune parameters in murine OVA-induced allergic diarrhea..." and "N. sativa seed extract seems to be a promising candidate for nutritional interventions in humans with food allergy." REF - 'Nigella sativa (black cumin) seed extract alleviates symptoms of allergic diarrhea in mice, involving opioid receptors'

Black seed oil also aids the immune system when it comes to protecting against radioactivity! "Our results strongly recommend Nigella sativa oil as a promising natural radioprotective agent against immunosuppressive and oxidative effects of ionizing radiation." REF - 'Radioprotective effects of black seed (Nigella sativa) oil against hemopoietic damage and immunosuppression in gamma-irradiated rats'

Remember near the start of this book I listed the active constituents of black seed oil and the most prevalent and researched is Thymoquinone. Most research focuses on Thymoquinone, but this next research paper studied both Thymoquinone and nigellone. In this study on mucus clearance and trachea contractions, the nigellone won out over Thymoquinone. "In conclusion, this study provides evidence for an antispasmodic effect and an increase in mucociliary clearance for nigellone but not for Thymoquinone. Altogether the data indicate that nigellone but not Thymoquinone may be useful in the treatment of different respiratory diseases." REF - 'The effect of nigellone and Thymoquinone on inhibiting trachea contraction and mucociliary clearance'

So, it seems that black seed oil wins again, this time against colds and flu.

In 1999, at the 1st International Conference on Scientific Miracles of Qu-ran and Sunnah, the conference that has been accused of being bias in digging up scientific research merely to support the claims made in the Qur'an, made sure to mention at this inaugural event the supreme healing powers of black seed oil. After all, it is described in that holy book as the remedy for all ailments except death, so why wouldn't they tout its merits at the very first opportunity? There's no link nor book reference I could find on this pre-internet dated conference, though it is referenced by science papers the world over.

Would you believe that there has also been research done on the avian influenza virus H5N1 using black seed oil as an alternative adjuvant in the chicken vaccine? Remember, an adjuvant is a substance that helps to activate the immune system, otherwise known as immunostimulants. They were checking out the immunostimulant effect of the black seed oil and got some fabulous results, "The H5-DNA vaccine with Nigella sativa oil adjuvant induced potent cell-mediated immune response in chickens reached up to 86% phagocytic percent and 0.5 lymphocyte proliferation at 14th day post vaccination." REF - 'Nigella sativa oil as an immunostimulant adjuvant in H5 based DNA vaccine of H5N1 avian influenza virus'

Interestingly, I also found a link to a paper called 'Effects of Nigella sativa on immune responses and pathogenesis of avian influenza (H9N2) virus in turkeys', however, that paper had been retracted, "...due to an existing conflict of interest and ethical issues in the contents of the article. The corresponding author has voluntarily requested this retraction for the betterment of science and under ethical considerations." That seems like a fascinating enigma.

References

'A review on therapeutic potential of Nigella sativa: A miracle herb'
Majdalawieh AF, Hmaidan R, Carr RI. J Ethnopharmacol. 2010;131(2):268–275.

'Evaluation of immunomodulatory effect of three herbal plants growing in Egypt'
https://www.ncbi.nlm.nih.gov/pubmed/20507215 (as accessed 19 June 2018).

'Nigella sativa (black cumin) seed extract alleviates symptoms of allergic diarrhea in mice, involving opioid receptors'
https://www.ncbi.nlm.nih.gov/pmc/articles/PMC3387213/ (as accessed 20 June 2018).

'Radioprotective effects of black seed (Nigella sativa) oil against hemopoietic damage and immunosuppression in gamma-irradiated rats'
https://www.sigmaaldrich.com/catalog/papers/20105084 (as accessed 20 June 2018).

'The effect of nigellone and Thymoquinone on inhibiting trachea contraction and mucociliary clearance'
https://www.ncbi.nlm.nih.gov/pubmed/18219598 (as accessed 20 June 2018).

'Nigella sativa oil as an immunostimulant adjuvant in H5

based DNA vaccine of H5N1 avian influenza virus'
Global Veterinaria 10(6):663-668 · January 2013

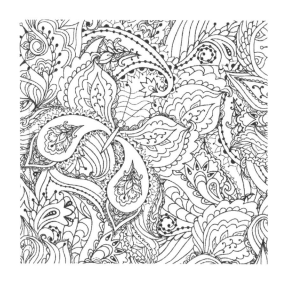

Chapter 22 – Inflammation

Black seed oil is a fantastic anti-inflammatory. In fact, that's why I first bought it; to ease my inflamed back. I have trialled myself on 7 different brands of black seed oil during the last year or so and it's been the life blessing for me that the Ancients told us about.

What is Inflammation?

Inflammation is one way that our bodies tell us that something is wrong and needs our attention. This is your immune system doing a good job. When inflammation occurs, this is a good sign to give your immune system a boost with black seed oil or other immune boosters. As you will see, the black seed oil is fabulous at aiding inflammation in the human body.

The Research

In randomized double-blind, placebo-controlled clinical trials, black cumin seed oil has proven itself to be a fantastic anti-inflammatory.

One study even goes so far as to tout Nigella sativa as a "...potential cure for inflammatory disorders" REF - 'Thymoquinone: potential cure for inflammatory disorders and cancer'

Even in cadmium-induced lung injury, black cumin seed oil mitigates the negative symptoms.

In regards to the inflammation caused by asthma, "Nigella sativa showed a statistically significant improvement in ACT and blood eosinophils count." REF - 'Mitigation of cadmium-induced lung injury by Nigella sativa oil.'

Rheumatoid arthritis sufferers can benefit from the healing power of these seeds too:

"This study indicates that Nigella sativa could improve inflammation and reduce oxidative stress in patients with rheumatoid arthritis. It is suggested that Nigella sativa may be a beneficial adjunct therapy in this population of patients." -

A study on rats found that both the black seed oil volatile compound and Thymoquinone were found to have a "significant dose-dependent anti-inflammatory effect" REF -

'A study of the anti-inflammatory activity of Nigella sativa L. and Thymoquinone in rats'

Yet another study on rats was done showing a reduction in inflammation markers on spinal cord ischemia-reperfusion injury. Malondialdehyde and nitric oxide oxidative markers were reduced, as were cytokines. REF - 'Neuroprotective effects of Thymoquinone against spinal cord ischemia-reperfusion injury by attenuation of inflammation, oxidative stress, and apoptosis'

So, as you can see, there is a huge amount of research on the anti-inflammatory benefits of the not-so-humble black cumin seed.

I highly recommend black seed oil, mainly for the pain relief it offers me through its anti-inflammatory properties.

References
'A study of the anti-inflammatory activity of Nigella sativa L. and Thymoquinone in rats'
https://www.researchgate.net/publication/282199860 (as accessed 18 June 2018)

'Thymoquinone: potential cure for inflammatory disorders and cancer'
https://www.ncbi.nlm.nih.gov/pubmed/22005518 (as accessed 18 June 2018).
'Mitigation of cadmium-induced lung injury by Nigella

sativa oil.' https://www.ncbi.nlm.nih.gov/pubmed/27696167 (as accessed 18 June 2018).

'Neuroprotective effects of Thymoquinone against spinal cord ischemia-reperfusion injury by attenuation of inflammation, oxidative stress, and apoptosis' http://thejns.org/doi/10.3171/2015.10.SPINE15612 (as accessed 18 June 2018).

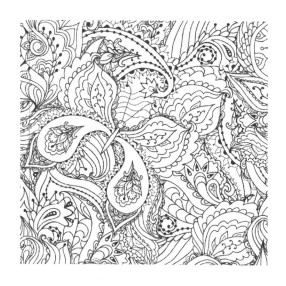

Chapter 23 – Ischemic Heart Disease

The word ischemic means reduced blood supply and when it's followed by the word heart, we are talking about reduced blood flow to the heart. Otherwise known as coronary artery disease, ischemic heart disease refers to a group of diseases including angina, myocardial infarction, and sudden cardiac death.

What is Ischemic Heart Disease?
Ischemic heart disease usually develops when cholesterol particles in the blood lodge on the walls of the arteries that supply blood to the heart. Plaque deposits end up forming and narrowing the arteries and, eventually, blocks the flow of blood. This (usually) gradual decrease in blood flow reduces the amount of oxygen supplied to the heart muscle,

slowly but surely stopping the heart from doing its job.

The Research

During a study in 2017, researchers used 15 rats divided into 3 groups; those fed black seed oil (800 mg/Kg daily), another group was put on an exercise treadmill for 2 hours per day and the final group was the control group. The researchers found, "NS effect on coronary angiogenesis needs to be explored further as it might lead to a new promising preventive and therapeutic agent of the ischemic heart disease." REF - 'Coronary angiogenic effect of long-term administration of Nigella sativa'

In another rat study, this time in 2015 using a daily dose of 20 mg/kg/day, researchers found, "Treatment with TMQ prevented the depletion of endogenous antioxidants and myocyte injury marker enzymes and inhibited lipid peroxidation as well as reducing the levels of proinflammatory cytokines. TMQ pre-treatment also reduced myonecrosis, edema, and infiltration of inflammatory cells and showed preservation of cardiomyocytes histoarchitecture. The present study results demonstrate that TMQ exerts a cardioprotective effect by mitigating oxidative stress, augmenting endogenous antioxidants, and maintaining structural integrity. The results of the present study indicate that TMQ may serve as an excellent agent alone or as an adjuvant to prevent the onset and progression of myocardial injury." REF - 'Thymoquinone Protects against Myocardial Ischemic Injury by Mitigating Oxidative Stress and Inflammation'

Dyslipidemia being an established risk factor for ischemic heart disease, this review study provides some more hope for black seed oil in treating this disease. "...different preparations of NS including seed powder (100 mg-20 g daily), seed oil (20-800 mg daily), Thymoquinone (3.5-20 mg daily), and seed extract (methanolic extract especially), were shown to reduce plasma levels of total cholesterol, low-density lipoprotein cholesterol (LDL-C) and triglycerides, but the effect on high-density lipoprotein cholesterol (HDL-C) was not significant." REF - 'Ameliorative effects of Nigella sativa on dyslipidemia'

References

'Coronary angiogenic effect of long-term administration of Nigella sativa'
https://www.ncbi.nlm.nih.gov/pmc/articles/PMC5470270/ (as accessed 21 June 2018).

'Thymoquinone Protects against Myocardial Ischemic Injury by Mitigating Oxidative Stress and Inflammation'
https://www.ncbi.nlm.nih.gov/pmc/articles/PMC4458551/ (as accessed 21 June 2018).

'Ameliorative effects of Nigella sativa on dyslipidemia'
https://www.ncbi.nlm.nih.gov/pubmed/26134064 (as accessed 21 June 2018)/

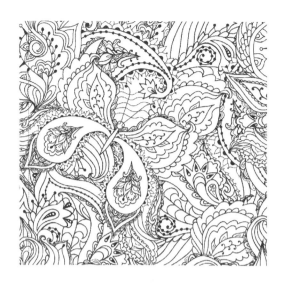

Chapter 24 - Lupus

Otherwise known as Systemic lupus erythematosus, this is an autoimmune disease in which the immune system inappropriately attacks healthy tissue in many parts of the body, causing all sorts of damage along the way. If you have lupus then you are probably looking for some relief that big pharma can't or won't offer you.

What is Lupus?
This is a chronic, inflammatory autoimmune condition that affects each victim differently.

The Research
Again, there isn't much published research on this subject. Instead, we have to look at the mechanism of lupus and see if we can find an inroad there. Lupus is an autoimmune

condition, so it makes sense to figure out if black seed can help with immune system issues. And, yes, it does. For information on this, please see the chapter on colds/flu.

In 2015, Egyptian researchers stated, "We noticed a significant increase in the levels of SOD and GSH in SLE patients following treatment with Nigella sativa and vitamin E in comparison to pre-treatment levels (P<0.001 for both). While the levels of IL-10, MDA, NO, iNOS decreased significantly following treatment (P<0.001 for all). Conclusion: The improvement of selected oxidative and nitrosative biomarkers and SLEDAI score favours antioxidant therapy in SLE." REF - 'Effect of Nigella Sativa and Vitamin E on Some Oxidative / Nitrosative Biomarkers in Systemic Lupus Erythematosus Patients'

References
'Effect of Nigella Sativa and Vitamin E on Some Oxidative / Nitrosative Biomarkers in Systemic Lupus Erythematosus Patients' Life Science Journal 2015;12(7) (as accessed 24 June 2018).

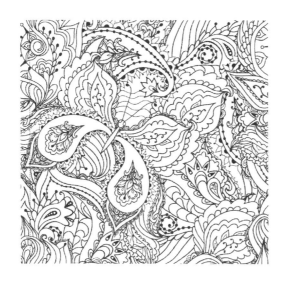

Chapter 25 – Lyme

"In the fullness of time, the mainstream handling of chronic Lyme disease will be viewed as one of the most shameful episodes in the history of medicine because elements of academic medicine, elements of government, and virtually the entire insurance industry have colluded to deny a disease. This has resulted in needless suffering of many individuals who deteriorate and sometimes die for lack of timely application of treatment or denial of treatment beyond some arbitrary duration"

- Dr Kenneth Liegner, Physician since 1988

Lyme (Lyme borreliosis) seems to be a mysterious kind of disease to Australians that DON'T have it because we have been told for decades that it doesn't exist here. I find that a bizarre claim by the 'authorities' because it's plain to see the extent of it when you talk to sufferers. Then there's this little tidbit from the government, "While there is no evidence that Lyme disease is caused by Australian ticks, there may be other infections carried by Australian ticks which may cause an infection which is similar to Lyme disease. These infections remain poorly characterised." (If it smells like shit and tastes like shit, then it's probably shit, ahem!)

Note the continuation of the sneaky language, "Although locally-acquired Lyme disease cannot be ruled out, there is little evidence that it occurs in Australia." Remember, little evidence and zero evidence are not the same thing. If they were in possession of zero evidence, that's what they'd state. REF – NSW Health 'Lyme disease fact sheet'

This is also from our government health department, "Position Statement: Lyme disease in Australia. Classical Lyme disease is an infectious disease that can be transmitted to humans if bitten by a tick carrying Borrelia burgdorferi sensu lato. In Australia, this organism has yet to be identified in Australian ticks or any another vector that could transmit a disease to humans. It is for this reason that the Australian Government does not support the diagnosis of locally acquired Lyme disease in Australia." REF - 'Position Statement: Lyme disease in Australia'

What is Lyme?
On an Australian government website, it tells us that Lyme

disease "...is a tick-borne infection caused by bacteria in the Borrelia burgdorferi sensu lato group.

The first symptom is usually a characteristic pink or red rash that starts as a small red spot that gradually spreads in a much larger circle with a characteristic bulls-eye appearance called erythema migrans."

The Research

Yet again, there is little to zero direct black seed oil and Lyme disease research, so again, we go down the rabbit hole to the symptoms associated with the disease.

For starters, Thymoquinone inhibits the NF-kB group of proteins. These proteins are associated with inflammation and autoimmune disorders." REF - 'Macrophage polarization comes of age'

A boosted white blood cell count is essential to your immune response in the fight against Lyme, and black seed oil is a definite assistant there too. In 2009, researchers found, "... a preventive effect of Thymoquinone, one constituent of N. sativa, on tracheal responsiveness and inflammatory cells of lung lavage of sensitized guinea pigs which was comparable or even greater than that of the inhaled steroid." REF - 'The Effect of Thymoquinone, the Main Constituent of Nigella sativa on Tracheal Responsiveness and White Blood Cell Count in Lung Lavage of Sensitized Guinea Pigs'

References

NSW Health 'Lyme disease fact sheet'
http://www.health.nsw.gov.au/Infectious/factsheets/Pages/lyme_disease.aspx (as accessed 25 June 2018).

'Position Statement: Lyme disease in Australia'
http://www.health.gov.au/internet/main/publishing.nsf/Content/ohp-lyme-disease.htm/$File/Posit-State-Lyme-June18.pdf

'Macrophage polarization comes of age'
https://www.ncbi.nlm.nih.gov/pubmed/16226499 (as accessed 25 June 2018).

'The Effect of Thymoquinone, the Main Constituent of Nigella sativa on Tracheal Responsiveness and White Blood Cell Count in Lung Lavage of Sensitized Guinea Pigs'
https://www.researchgate.net/publication/26771192 (as accessed 25 June 2018).

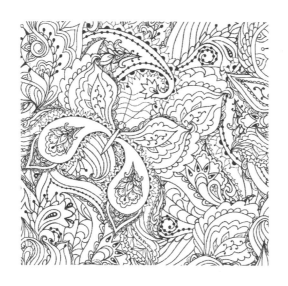

Chapter 26 - Menopause

Hello, Ladies! My name is Pixie and I'm a menopause survivor! How did I do it? With black seed oil and yogahh (no typo!). Add to that the beginning of my mindfulness training and no one got hurt. Go me!

What is Menopause?

Simply put, menopause is the end of menstrual cycles. With this comes a whole new hormonal level and body changes to adjust to. Never mind, we've been doing this our entire lives, Lovelies. Embrace this time of life with as much grace as you can muster, but, don't worry if you lose your shit occasionally because it happens to the best of us. Good luck!

The Research

A group of researchers in Malaysia did a trial on a group of

30 menopausal women. They were split into 2 groups and 1 group was given 1 x 1 gram per day of black seed in capsule form. Their conclusion after 2 months was, "These results suggested that treatment with N. sativa exert a protective effect by improving lipid profile and blood glucose which are in higher risk to be elevated during menopausal period." REF - 'Protective Effects of Nigella sativa on Metabolic Syndrome in Menopausal Women'

In the official journal of the International Society for Complementary Medicine Research (ISCMR), there is a study from 2014 that states, "Nigella sativa reverses osteoporosis in ovariectomized rats, which could be attributed to its high content of unsaturated fatty acids as well as its antioxidant and anti-inflammatory properties." That's protection for your bones right there! REF - 'Nigella Sativa reverses osteoporosis in ovariectomized rats'

Then there's this conclusion from another research article, "The finding indicated the probable beneficial role for N. sativa in the treatment of postmenopausal symptoms and possibility of using N. sativa as an alternative to hormone replacement therapy (HRT) for post menopause in humans." - REF - 'Effect of Nigella sativa on reproductive system in experimental menopause rat model'
There is more menopause research in the estrogen chapter.

References
'Protective Effects of Nigella sativa on Metabolic Syndrome

in Menopausal Women' -
http://journals.tbzmed.ac.ir/APB/Manuscript/APB-4-29.pdf
(as accessed 24 June 2018).

'Nigella Sativa reverses osteoporosis in ovariectomized rats'
https://bmccomplementalternmed.biomedcentral.com/article
s/10.1186/1472-6882-14-22 (as accessed 24 June 2018).

'Effect of Nigella sativa on reproductive system in
experimental menopause rat model'
http://ajp.mums.ac.ir/article_6079_ec23387ad355c8703ce9358
676f94559.pdf (as accessed 24 June 2018).

Menopause

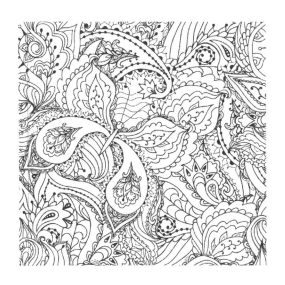

Chapter 27 – Nausea

Try as I did, I couldn't find any research that has been done on black cumin seed and nausea. What I did find were many, many anecdotes about how nausea was cured by taking black cumin seed oil orally. The links to these anecdotes are in the references section below.

What is Nausea?
That icky feeling in the belly like it's churning is the feeling of nausea. Usually, it goes away after a few minutes, but some poor souls put up with this awful feeling for a lot longer.

I guess because nausea isn't a life-threatening disease or disorder it doesn't get a scientific mention. Fair enough. I did go through the online science and medical journals and really couldn't find anything specific to link nausea and black seed oil.

References

http://projectavalon.net/forum4/showthread.php?38248-Nigella-sativa-Black-Cumin-Black-Seed

http://conscioushealthnaturaltherapy.weebly.com/research---nigella-sativa.html

http://articles.mercola.com/sites/articles/archive/2016/01/25/black-cumin-seed-benefits.aspx

http://www.greenmedinfo.com/blog/cumin-essential-oil-offers-relief-ibs-clinical-study

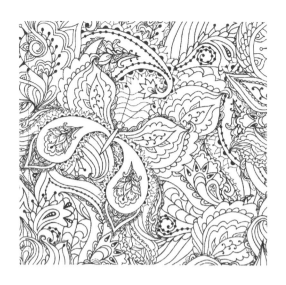

Chapter 28 – Oil vs. Powder

I believe that it comes down to personal preference. Yes, the raw seeds, chewed into a powder are more nutritious and have more activated Thymoquinone in them. However, if you're like me, you can't actually hold them in your mouth that long!

What is Oil and Powder?
Oils are greasy and when ingesting, you wash them down with orange juice or a hot drink, never cold. Powders are meant to be mixed with water to ingest or swallowed in capsule form. Oil capsules are also available.

Nothing is lost in the making of the black seed oil because it's cold pressed. This leaves just the pure oil.

The research

Some people swear by the chewing of seeds method, but I just can't do it. You can get the oil in capsule form if you want to take it internally. The regular dosage is 1000mg per day, taken in 2 capsules, but as always, follow the directions on the bottle or packet.

The Strength Issue

1 teaspoon of oil = 2.5 teaspoons of seeds, on average. So, from an economic point of view, it's much cheaper to take the oils. Sometimes it may be more convenient to use the powder? I don't know as I've always used the oils for their potency.

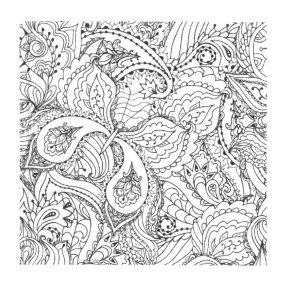

Chapter 29 – Organic Suppliers

Have you ever read a book with a website link, only to go to that link and find the site has changed or is no longer on that domain name? I have, lots of times. It's as annoying as it is unnecessary. Therefore, I am going to provide you with ONE solitary website, mine, that will still be up and running 20 years from now… and longer!

I will tell you that, yes, I do get a small commission from your purchase. I do this to fund my research. As you may know, my research is NON-pharma related and, as such, doesn't attract much funding (to say the least!). In addition, if you know me at all, you know that I am above all else, honest. There are some products that I could have recommended but they just aren't up to scratch. The black seed oils I do recommend are a little more expensive than some others, however, not only can you not put a price on your good health, but you are also supporting the good work that I do in regards to bringing back natural health to the world! Remember the old adage, 'You get what you pay for'? Well, that doesn't apply to all things but I'm sure you can agree that it does apply to most. Black seed oil is no different.

The very best thing about me sending you to my own website instead of a bunch of other links is that I am committed to always bringing you, dear Reader, the most up to date information. Therefore, when you visit my site, the black seed oil that I recommend may have changed IF I find a better one. Including links here limits your updates!

Here is my site link with my most up to date black seed oil recommendations;
www.detoxnaturalliving.com/blackseedoilmasterguide.html

Thank you in advance for supporting my research mission to dig up the natural healing truth by purchasing through the links on my site.

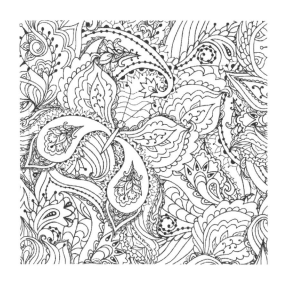

Chapter 30 – Parasites

Anthelmintic is the unusual word for an antiparasitic compound, and yes, you guessed it... Black seed oil is an anthelmintic!

What are Parasites?
A parasite, by definition, is an organism that lives on or in a host organism that it feeds off. Yes, some parasites live in happy co-existence with us humans, but others, particularly worms, we can live without. We, in modern times, struggle for a solution to de-worming ourselves from the constant contact with others, especially children. Like a lot of other modern 'remedies', the chemical cocktail required to kill worms can be quite toxic to the human body too. Remembering the ways of black seed oil is a blessing yet again when it comes to parasites like worms.

The Research

There is some research with regards to black seed oil being an antiparasitic compound with a few different types of parasites.

In 2014, researchers investigated the black seed ethanolic extract against Ascarissuum and had good results. "In conclusion, the black seeds (N. sativa) ethanolic extract had antihelminthic effect against A. suum." REF - 'In-Vitro Antihelminthic Effect of Ethanol Extract of Black Seeds (Nigella sativa) Against Ascaris suum'

Another study found that "Nigella sativa seeds were tested in vitro against Schistosoma mansoni miracidia, cercariae, and adult worms. Results indicate its strong biocidal effects against all stages of the parasite and also showed an inhibitory effect on the egg-laying of adult female worms" REF - 'Sativa seeds against Schistosoma mansoni different stages'

Helicobacter Pylori's last stand with black seed, "N. sativa seeds possess clinically useful anti-H. pylori activity, comparable to triple therapy." REF - 'Comparative study of Nigella Sativa and triple therapy in eradication of Helicobacter Pylori in patients with non-ulcer dyspepsia'

Fasciola hepatica and Fasciola gigantica are two species of parasite that mainly affect animals but humans are also known to be at risk of infection too. In India in 2017, the researchers found that both turmeric (curcumin) and Thymoquinone are effective at beating these parasites. "It is concluded that both the compounds understudy will decrease the detoxification ability of F. gigantica, while inhibition of CatL will significantly affect their virulence potential. Thus, both Thymoquinone and curcumin appeared to be promising anthelmintic compounds for further investigations." REF - 'Anthelmintic Potential of Thymoquinone and Curcumin on Fasciola gigantica'

References

'In-Vitro Antihelminthic Effect of Ethanol Extract of Black Seeds (Nigella sativa) Against Ascaris suum' - Procedia Chemistry Volume 13, 2014, Pages 181-185.

'Comparative study of Nigella Sativa and triple therapy in eradication of Helicobacter Pylori in patients with non-ulcer dyspepsia' https://www.ncbi.nlm.nih.gov/pubmed/20616418 (as accessed 22 June 2018).

'Anthelmintic Potential of Thymoquinone and Curcumin on Fasciola gigantica' http://journals.plos.org/plosone/article?id=10.1371/journal.pone.0171267 (as accessed 22 June 2018).

'Sativa seeds against Schistosoma mansoni different stages' - Mem Inst Oswaldo Cruz, Rio de Janeiro, Vol. 100(2): 205-211, April 2005.

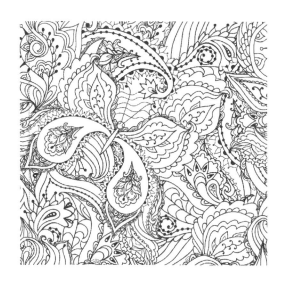

Chapter 31 – Pets

I don't know about you, but any and all natural therapies that I use on myself, I also apply to my dear dogga. In smaller amounts, of course! I also follow the very same protocol that I use and that starts with 1 drop and builds up slowly over time.

What is Pet Care with Black Seed Oil?
For those of you that view your pets as family (and they are!), you want the very best health care for them. If you are smart, that will usually only include natural substances.

In my research travels, I found a few different commercial canine and feline preparations that contained black seed so I feel pretty safe giving it to my pets.

The Research

I scoured the internet for research articles concerning black seed and dogs or cats and, truly, there's zero. So, it's up to us to figure it out for ourselves.

I use the black seed oil on my dogs. With each dog, I start with that 1 drop rubbed into the gum line. If there's no allergic reaction, then I start upping the dose a few drops at a time. After I have my dose, there is about 1ml left in the container and I rub it into their fur on their backs. There is usually an attempt to lick it off so it's not yukky to them. But, I put it in a spot where most of it will be inaccessible to lick-a-lot.

I apply black seed to the doggas for the enormous amount of health benefits it confers. I figure that if it's good for me, then it should be good for most mammals. In addition, I occasionally add a little to a few dog bikkies.

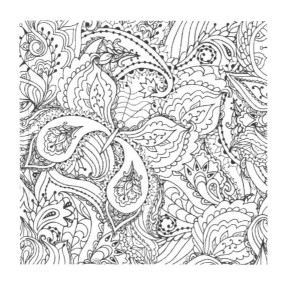

Chapter 32 – Pregnancy

This super oil has the potential to affect human pregnancies negatively by making the uterine walls contract. I think you will agree that is NOT a good idea, especially since that is what has to happen to push the baby out during labour!

What is Pregnancy?
You're kidding? You don't know?

The Research
Even though it is considered beneficial in animal studies, when it comes to humans, it seems that the black seed oil can "...affect the smooth muscle contractions of the uterus."

I've even seen suggestions that black seed can help prevent pregnancy. So, best to avoid, avoid, avoid, just like a lot of things during pregnancy.

Hang in there, it gets better in time. Enjoy your pregnancy with all the wonderful healing herbs that you ARE allowed instead!

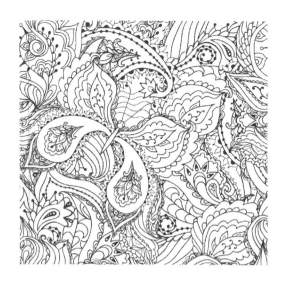

Chapter 33 – Staphylococcus

Otherwise known as methicillin-resistant staphylococcus aureus (MRSA), this is an infection that is rampant in hospitals. Sometimes referred to as Golden Staph. Note the word 'resistant' in its name? Yes, this is a tough infection to beat. This particular staph infection is 'resistant' to antibiotics, lots of different antibiotics. That's what makes it such a threat; the doctors have run out of prescribing options.

What is Staphylococcus?
Acquiring these infections is generally associated with invasive procedures, such as surgeries, intravenous tubing and artificial joints. This is because the infection can live on the skin.

Known as a 'genus of Gram-positive bacteria', it lives on the skin or in the nose or mouth. Spread with person to person contact, even though those that come in contact with a person that has staph won't usually get infected, however, open wound to open wound can result in infection (but who does that?!).

If this infection enters the bloodstream, it can be a serious problem, other than that, it's generally benign and doesn't cause any trouble until you have a wound.

Hand washing, hand washing, hand washing! ...will keep the chance of infection from staph low.

The Research
There is a growing body of evidence that black seed annoys the hell out of staphylococcus infections.

In 2008, researchers found that "The results indicated that N. sativa has an inhibitory effect on MRSA. This finding warrants the necessity of further investigation of this product of folk medicine." REF - 'Antibacterial activity of Nigella sativa against clinical isolates of methicillin-resistant Staphylococcus aureus.'

"Both the oil and extract showed remarkable dose-dependent antibacterial activity against the tested strains up to a dilution of 1:50 as evident from the zones of inhibition" and, "it may be concluded that Nigella sativa oil as well as extract are active against multidrug-resistant strains of

Coagulase-negative staphylococci and may be used, at least topically, in susceptible cases" REF - 'Antimicrobial activity of Black Cumin seeds (Nigella sativa) against multidrug-resistant strains of Coagulase-negative Staphylococci'

References

'Antibacterial activity of Nigella sativa against clinical isolates of methicillin-resistant Staphylococcus aureus.' https://www.ncbi.nlm.nih.gov/pubmed/19610522 (as accessed 23 June 2018).

'Antimicrobial activity of Black Cumin seeds (Nigella sativa) against multidrug-resistant strains of Coagulase Negative Staphylococci' https://www.academia.edu/179365 (as accessed 23 June 2018).

Staphylococcus

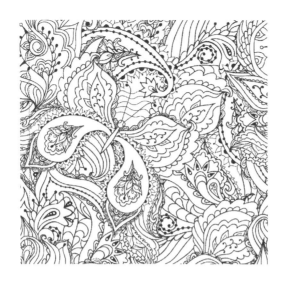

Chapter 34 – Thyroid

The American Thyroid Association says, about a thyroid study done on 47 Hashimoto's thyroiditis sufferers, "This study suggests that powdered black cumin may have beneficial effects on patients with Hashimoto's thyroiditis. However, this was only an 8-week study and more studies are needed to confirm whether this compound may help in the management of thyroid disorders"

What is the Thyroid?
With two hormones, triiodothyronine and thyroxine, the thyroid gland is the primary regulator of metabolism. The thyroid gland influences almost all of the metabolic processes in your body. Too much thyroid hormone and you will get hyperthyroidism. Not enough hormone production leads to hypothyroidism. There are a few other problems

that occur with the thyroid, but those are the main two and they can lead to all sorts of nasty complications.

The Research

While I could only find 2 research studies directly connecting black seed oil to thyroid problems, if we look to the causes of thyroid problems, we find things like autoimmune diseases, tumours – both benign and malignant –and inflammation. Earlier chapters of this book explain how black seed oil can help with all those health issues.

The first study was a double-blind, placebo-controlled trial of black seed on 40 participants suffering from Hashimoto's thyroiditis (most of which were women) and found that, "After 8 weeks of treatment (1 gram x 2 per day) participants in the Nigella group saw a significant reduction in all anthropometric values, while no significant change was seen in the placebo group.

Our data showed a potent beneficial effect of powdered Nigella sativa in improving thyroid status and anthropometric variables in patients with Hashimoto's thyroiditis." REF - 'The effects of Nigella sativa on thyroid function, serum vascular endothelial growth factor (VEGF)-1, nesfatin-1 and anthropometric features in patients with Hashimoto's thyroiditis: a randomized controlled trial'

The second study investigated the effects of black seed on the thyroid hormones, triiodothyronine and thyroxine, in diabetic rats. They found "The mean concentration of serum T3 was significantly ($p<0.001$) decreased in animals of diabetic (control) group as compared to that of animals in the control group. However, in animals of the NS-treated group, mean serum T3 concentration was significantly ($p<0.001$) increased compared to the diabetic group." REF - 'Effect of Nigella sativa on serum concentrations of thyroid hormones and thyroid stimulating hormone in alloxan-induced diabetic albino rats'

References

'The effects of Nigella sativa on thyroid function, serum vascular endothelial growth factor (VEGF)-1, nesfatin-1 and anthropometric features in patients with Hashimoto's thyroiditis: a randomized controlled trial' - BMC Complement Altern Med. 2016;16:471.

'Effect of Nigella sativa on serum concentrations of thyroid hormones and thyroid stimulating hormone in alloxan-induced diabetic albino rats'
https://www.thefreelibrary.com/EFFECT+OF+NIGELLA+SA TIVA+ON+SERUM+CONCENTRATIONS+OF+THYROID+ HORMONES...-a0484653376

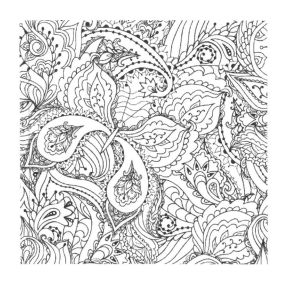

Chapter 35 – Tumours - Benign

There are 2 types of cancer; benign (non-dangerous) and malignant (dangerous). In this chapter, I will discuss the benign tumours (see the earlier chapter about malignant cancers).

When I apply a little logic here, if black cumin seed oil positively treats malignant cancers, and it does, then surely the same amazing results can be had for benign cancers?

What is a Benign Tumour?
There are a few different types of benign tumours and the names of them correspond to the body part affected. The different types are; adenomas, meningiomas, fibromas (fibroids), papillomas, lipomas, nevi, myomas, hemangiomas, neuromas, and osteochondromas.

The Research

There isn't a lot of research on this subject, but when black cumin treatment is having positive effects on malignant cancers, then you can be reasonably sure that it will have a similar effect on benign tumours too.

One research article states, "Pre-treatment of TQ in the PCO rat model induced significant restoration of normal physio-molecular behaviour of the ovary, such as reduced cysts formation, increased ovulation rate, and normalization of key ovarian factors." REF - 'Implication of Thymoquinone as a remedy for polycystic ovary in rats'

In a review research paper in 2010, it states, "TQ has anti-inflammatory effects, and it inhibits tumour cell proliferation through modulation of apoptosis signalling, inhibition of angiogenesis, and cell cycle arrest." REF - 'Review on molecular and therapeutic potential of Thymoquinone in cancer.'

Another research paper states, "... TQ interferes with polyp progression in ApcMin mice through induction of tumour-cell specific apoptosis and by modulating Wnt signalling..." - 'Thymoquinone attenuates tumour growth in ApcMin mice by interference with Wnt-signalling.' https://www.ncbi.nlm.nih.gov/pubmed/23668310 (as accessed 2 June 2018).

References

'Implication of Thymoquinone as a remedy for polycystic ovary in rats'
https://www.ncbi.nlm.nih.gov/pubmed/26510692 (as accessed 2 June 2018).

'Review on molecular and therapeutic potential of Thymoquinone in cancer.'
https://www.ncbi.nlm.nih.gov/pubmed/20924969 (as accessed 2 June 2018).

'Thymoquinone attenuates tumour growth in ApcMin mice by interference with Wnt-signalling.'
https://www.ncbi.nlm.nih.gov/pubmed/23668310 (as accessed 2 June 2018).

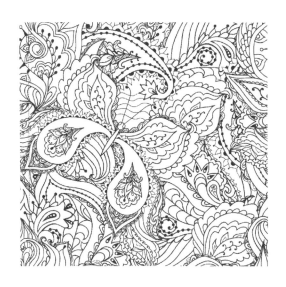

36 – Weight Loss

Again, not a lot of research has been done on this subject, and I found most of the research with regards to weight loss with black cumin seed in diabetic studies.

What is Weight Loss?
We become overweight for so many different reasons, but with willpower (there's no getting around that one, sorry!) and a few herbal helpers like black seed and exercise, you can get rid of all the fat you want. I know this because I lived it after gaining and losing 40kg (88lb!). That's a story for another day.

As always, consult your health professional first, especially if you are in the obese range (<30% body fat).

The Research

There was a study done on menopausal women that showed good results of weight loss with black seed oil.

"Nigella Sativa [black cumin] showed a significant weight loss and reduced waist circumference with a mild reduction in fasting blood sugar, triglycerides and low-density lipoprotein levels." This was achieved with a dose of 1.5 gm powder of black cumin seed oil (split into two capsules) that was given twice a day for three months. - REF - 'Nigella sativa (black seed) is an effective herbal remedy for every disease except death – a Prophetic statement which modern scientists confirm unanimously: A review'

In the next study, there is some more hope for black seed oil in weight loss with these statements, "...in the treatment group, complaints related to central obesity disappeared in the first week, very significant reduction of body weight, waist circumference, and systolic blood pressure..." and "It is suggested that a larger dose and longer duration of NS consumption will give better results." REF - 'Efficacy of Nigella sativa on serum free testosterone and metabolic disturbances in central obese male.'

Another Black Cumin Weight Loss Study Result

In a randomized, double-blind controlled clinical trial, it was found that "NS (Nigella sativa) oil concurrent with a low-calorie diet decreased weight... in obese women." REF -

Yet another study showing good results for the 50 obese female participants. The abstract states "N.sativa oil concurrent with a low-calorie diet decreased weight and increased SOD levels in obese women" REF - 'Oxidative Stress Responses to Nigella sativa Oil Concurrent with a Low-Calorie Diet in Obese Women: A Randomized, Double-Blind Controlled Clinical Trial.'

I hope you have figured out by now that, alongside a healthy intake of food, black cumin seed can help you with your weight loss.

References

'Nigella sativa (black seed) is an effective herbal remedy for every disease except death – a Prophetic statement which modern scientists confirm unanimously: A review' http://www.netjournals.org/pdf/AMPR/2016/2/16-008.pdf (as accessed 27 June 2018). http://www.academicjournals.org/jmpr/PDF/pdf2011/18April/Parhizkar%20et%20al.pdf

Efficacy of Nigella sativa on serum free testosterone and metabolic disturbances in central obese male.' Available from: https://www.ncbi.nlm.nih.gov/pubmed/20724766/ as accessed 27 Jan 2018).

'Oxidative Stress Responses to Nigella sativa Oil Concurrent with a Low-Calorie Diet in Obese Women: A Randomized, Double-Blind Controlled Clinical Trial.' Available from:

https://www.ncbi.nlm.nih.gov/pubmed/26179113 (as accessed 26 Jan 2018).

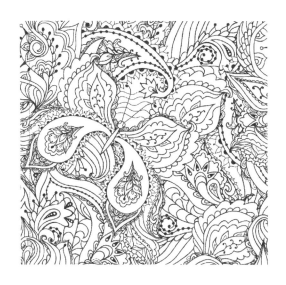

Chapter 37 – With Raw Honey

I'm about to introduce you to one of the most healing combinations that we have; black cumin and raw honey. And, yes, indeed, I have some research papers to back up what healers have known for millennia; these 2 compounds are a superior team to anything man-made.

What is Raw Honey?
Temperature and texture are the two definers of what separates honey from raw honey. If the honey is not heated beyond the point of pasteurization, then it's defined as raw.

The Research
Inside the hive, the bees take care of the temperature of the honey by using the collective body temperature heat which consequently warms their honey while they work. The

inside temperature of an active beehive is about 95ºF (35ºC). At that temperature, the honey is stable and still alive or 'raw', meaning that the enzymes in honey that give it the nutritional and beneficial qualities are alive and intact. As long as the temperature of the honey never significantly rises past 95ºF/35ºC, it's raw honey.

The health benefits from raw honey come from the synergistic effect of:
- 22 amino acids
- 27 minerals and
- 5,000 enzymes

There is evidence that the raw honey and black cumin combination is killing cancer cells in rat studies. REF - 'Inhibition of methylnitrosourea (MNU) induced oxidative stress and carcinogenesis by orally administered bee honey and Nigella grains in Sprague Dawley rats.'

Minerals in Raw Honey
Iron, potassium, zinc, selenium, phosphorous, magnesium and calcium.

Vitamins in Raw Honey
Vitamin B6, thiamin, riboflavin, pantothenic acid and niacin

Black Cumin Oil with Raw Honey
This combination is one of the most healing superfoods known to man! The list of ailments that do NOT get positively affected by the addition of black seed oil and

honey is surely shorter than the list that it does assist?!
The benefits of mixing these two superfood compounds is synergistic (greater than the sum of the two).

When reading research papers for hours on end, the expression "100%" jumps out at you and this is the number that slapped me when looking at black seed and raw honey combo research. The 100% refers to "Nigella sativa given orally protected against MNU-induced oxidative stress and carcinogenesis by 80% whereas honey and N. sativa seed together protected 100%" - REF 'Dermatological effects of Nigella sativa' https://www.sciencedirect.com/science/article/pii/S23522410 15000286#b0235 (as accessed 10 June 2018).

For an even healthier health-punch-in-the-guts, try adding some raw garlic to the black seed and honey concoction!

Honey contains floral flavonoids, which, when entering the body, immediately increase the antioxidant levels within cells. The honey goes on a scavenger hunt for oxidants and also stops the destruction of collagen in the body.

What's the Difference Between Raw Honey and Honey?
The difference here is HUGE. If it's called just 'honey' then it's usually been processed, removing most to ALL particles. Most of the goodness is filtered out of raw honey to make it into that clear stuff you see at the supermarket.

Most of the goodness that is removed is comprised of the enzymes!

Find a local supplier of your raw honey and ignore the clear stuff because the health benefits just aren't the same as the opaque types of honey.

Dosage

Black cumin seed oil is a maximum dosage of 1 teaspoon x 3 daily. Raw honey can be pretty much consumed at will, just don't go all honey bear on it, ahem! And if you want to add a clove of fresh, raw garlic to each teaspoon of black cumin and honey, that's an extra dose of an immune booster.

References

'Inhibition of methylnitrosourea (MNU) induced oxidative stress and carcinogenesis by orally administered bee honey and Nigella grains in Sprague Dawley rats.' Mabrouk et al., 2004. https://www.researchgate.net/publication/11075109 (as accessed 26 Jan 2018).

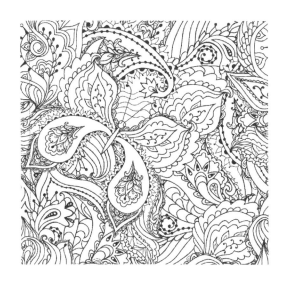

Conclusion

If you have read from cover to cover; great effort! Black cumin seed, especially the oil, is truly a wonder substance, eh!? I could hardly believe this list of conditions that it aids and the number of chemical compounds in it are beyond compare in the Natural world!

Keep this book as a reference guide and get yourself some great quality black seed oil, today. Seriously, this is a must-have item in any natural medicine cabinet.

I love this oil so much that I pretty much want to bathe in it, LOL!

Always Remember...

...nothing works all alone. Everything and everyone has a natural equilibrium that is affected by the total synergy of everything, including feeding your mind, body AND spirit.

If you live your life on the 'dark side' allowing negative emotions like envy, fear and hate to rule you...if you don't pay attention and be mindful of what you put in your mouth, on your skin and surround yourself with...but eat black cumin seeds, don't expect to be cured of what ails you, any time soon.

"Whether you think you can or think you can't, you're right" - Henry Ford. There is much truth in that quote, and I firmly believe that EVERYTHING is PERSPECTIVE.

The example of 2 identical people living identical lives, but 1 is happy and 1 is depressed is the best way to point out the difference that thinking can have on your general feeling of well-being.

Have you ever noticed that happy people stay relatively happy and that angry, sad people stay that way too? This happens for a number of reasons, but it is most important to note that by changing your thinking patterns, you can CHANGE YOUR LIFE! (I'm living proof!)

"Happy people are happy with what they have, in that moment. Just join those moments up for maximum happiness"

Conclusion

Make peace within YOU, then the world. Only then can you best help your body with healthy natural remedies like black cumin and raw honey mixtures. If you give your body what it needs, it can heal, boost the immune system and, in turn, fight off any invaders

When you balance the body, it has everything it needs to heal itself.

Even healthy bodies are well supported by a daily dose of this amazing little black cumin seed. You can cook with it, chew the seeds or take the oil. It's all good. Just remember to check the contraindications and with your health care provider. Ask them questions like, 'Have you done any research on black cumin seed as a natural therapy?'

I hope this book has served you well and I wish you an easy and enlightening trip on your natural health journey.

The last word must go to Zeba Farooqui, an environmental toxicology Research Scholar at Aligarh Muslim University, "Further research both in human and in animal models are urgently required to explore the mechanisms of action of the active ingredients of N. sativa seed, in particular TQ, in health and diseases at the cellular and molecular levels."

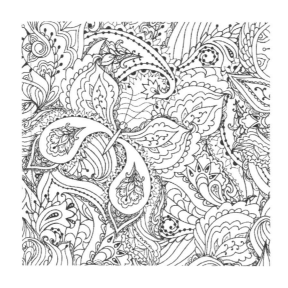

Other Black Seed Oil References

Indian Medicinal Plants: A Compendium of 500 Species - Warrier PK, Nambiar VPK, Ramankutty. Chennai: Orient Longman Pvt Ltd; 2004

Yarnell E, Abascal K.- 'Nigella sativa: holy herb of the Middle East'

Indian Medicinal Plants: A Compendium of 500 Species - Warrier PK, Nambiar VPK, Ramankutty. Chennai: Orient Longman Pvt Ltd; 2004

Database of Ayurveda Herbs - http://www.gbv.de/dms/bs/toc/387748814.pdf

Made in the USA
Middletown, DE
22 December 2021